# Incurable Us

## Why the Best Medical Research Does Not Make It into Clinical Practice

T0204916

### K. P. STOLLER, MD
**FOREWORD BY VERA SHARAV**

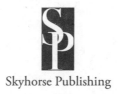

Skyhorse Publishing

Copyright © 2016 by Kenneth Paul Stoller
First paperback edition 2024
Foreword copyright © 2024 by Vera Sharav

Visit our website at www.skyhorsepublishing.com.

10 9 8 7 6 5 4 3 2 1

Library of Congress Cataloging-in-Publication Data is available on file.

Cover design by David Ter-Avanesyan
Cover image from Getty Images

Paperback ISBN: 978-1-5107-7494-0

Printed in the United States of America

This book is dedicated to my son Galen, for had he remained on Earth, I know he would be telling the truth to everyone he could, for first and foremost he was and still is a truth seeker.

*Temperate, sincere, and intelligent inquiry and discussion are only to be dreaded by the advocates of error. The truth need not fear them . . .*
—Dr. Benjamin Rush (1746–1813)
physician and Founding Father of the United States


*Was the government to prescribe to us our medicine and diet, our bodies would be in such keeping as our souls are now.*
—Thomas Jefferson (1743–1826)

# Table of Contents

**Foreword to the Revised Edition:** Never Again Is Now Global
                                   by Vera Sharav                    vii

**Introduction to the Revised Edition**                              xi

**Introduction to the First Edition**
*(Incurable Me)*, **Newly Revised**                                  xxxv

**Chapter 1:**        The House of Lyme                               1

**Chapter 2:**        Dementia: Are We All Getting Dicofo(o)l'ed?     29

**Chapter 3:**        Human Colony Collapse Disorder (Thanks for
                      all the Fish!)                                  55

**Chapter 4:**        Inflammatory Bowel Disease, or what a pile of . . .   68

**Chapter 5:**        Traumatic Brain Injury, Multiple Sclerosis, and
                      Hyperbaric Oxygen Therapy                       76

**Chapter 6:**        Mercury in Medicine: Quacks, Quackery,
                      and Quacksalber                                 91

**Chapter 7:**        The Religion of Jabism: A Special Chapter
                      on Vaccines                                     123

**Chapter 8:**        On Diagnosing and Treating Toxic/Infectious/
                      Immune Encephalopathy and Other Chronic Illness   144

**Chapter 9:**        The End of Addiction? *(New for Revised Edition)*   165

**Conclusion**                                                       171

**Notes**                                                            179

**Acknowledgments**                                                  203

**Index**                                                            204

*The right to search for truth implies also a duty. One must not conceal any part of what one has recognized to be true.*

—Albert Einstein (1879–1955); quote engraved in stone at the National Academy of Sciences in Washington, DC, home to the National Institutes of Health (NIH) and the Institute of Medicine (IOM)

# Foreword to the Revised Edition: Never Again Is Now Global

By Vera Sharav

In the first edition of *Incurable Us* (originally *Incurable Me*), Dr. Ken Stoller examined the corruption of medicine that is facilitated by a revolving door through which pharmaceutical company executives easily move to and from public health agencies that are supposed to regulate the industry. In this revised edition, Dr. Stoller examines the far more ominous, global perversion and weaponization of medicine; a perversion that threatens the very essence of a civilized society.

We are at a critical juncture in human history: a global totalitarian "regime takeover" threatens to eliminate our freedom of movement, our freedom to choose how to live our lives, and our human right to refuse to be injected with experimental genetically engineered medical interventions. The elimination of personal freedom will enslave us and destroy every aspect of our civilization.

The tragedy is that most people don't appreciate the threat confronting us. They don't comprehend the danger because they lack knowledge about the historic context. What's more, they have been methodically conditioned to trust and obey authority without questioning the rationale.

In January 1933, when Hitler gained political control, he declared a national emergency and swept aside constitutional government and personal freedom, as well as freedom of speech and the press. Under the Nazi regime expressed dissent was a crime.

As a survivor who has studied the history of the Holocaust, I know how a highly advanced, educated society and its academic, scientific, and cultural institutions can be perverted. I know what happens when moral norms and legal safeguards protecting individual rights are discarded and when segments of the population are demonized and disqualified as human beings. The entire fabric of a civilized society is torn apart.

Under the Nazi regime, the unthinkable was legitimized by the medical establishment. Doctors and nurses rationalized medical murder and genocide "for the greater good of society." Medical doctors actively participated in conceptualizing, initiating, and implementing mass murder policies under the guise of protecting public health.

The first medical murder victims were German infants and young children with disabilities. They were followed by disabled children of all ages, adults with mental or physical disabilities, and the elderly in nursing homes. Six German hospitals were transformed into medical killing centers.

As a survivor of that depraved genocidal regime, my mission is not only to remember, but to warn about foreboding current parallels. These include fomenting a state of fear maintained by incessant propaganda—just as the Nazis had fomented fear. The objective, then and now, was and is to psychologically condition people to be obedient and to follow government directives without question.

I shudder as I bear witness again: how the perversion of medicine and the weaponization of science and technology are paving the road to catastrophe once again. Today, we are confronted by an orchestrated, carefully planned, global demolition of personal freedom, human rights, human dignity, national sovereignty, and leaders who are accountable to the people they govern. This demolition is promoted under the guise of "protecting public health."

In March 2020, the World Health Organization declared a pandemic and governments around the globe issued a series of draconian directives and compulsory restrictions cloaked under the mantle of "protecting public health." These included lockdowns, quarantine, isolation of the elderly, closure of schools and houses of worship, and mandatory masks.

These destabilizing measures were crafted to promote a radical global political and financial agenda. Their immediate effect was to disrupt social interactions and to dismantle local economic activities. These uniform dictatorial measures and restrictions had nothing whatsoever to do with protecting public health. They are potent instruments of social and economic control. Those who questioned or challenged the need for onerous restrictions—even when these measures demonstrably caused harm—were denounced, ostracized, and accused of spreading the virus. Dissenters have been subjected to ridicule, as "spreaders of disinformation"—and thousands of people lost their jobs.

As Auschwitz survivor Primo Levi, a Jewish Polish chemist and author, observed: *"It happened, therefore, it can happen again; it can happen everywhere."*

The threat of genocide today is global. Technology has facilitated a global dictatorship by a band of global oligarchs who, like their Nazi predecessors, are deluded by their grandiosity. At the core of the assault on humanity—then and now—is the virulent ideology of eugenics. Although the terminology changed after the Nazi atrocities were made public, eugenics continues to infuse public health policies—as was demonstrated in March and April 2020. Government decrees in Western Europe, Australia, Canada, and the United States dictated medical treatment protocols and forbade hospitals to treat the elderly in care homes. Tens of thousands of elderly human beings were medically murdered.

The World Health Organization (WHO) is an unelected, unaccountable health agency that seeks to gain global control over our lives simply by asserting its right to declare a public health emergency. Two committees of the WHO have recently convened to discuss proposed amendments to the International Health Regulations (IHR 2005) and a new global Pandemic Treaty.

The immediate threat comes in a cluster of 307 proposed amendments to the IHR that would expand the definition of pandemics and health emergencies. They would replace evidence of "actual harm" with speculative "potential" for harm.

The director general of the WHO would be empowered "independently to declare emergencies" and would grant the WHO "control over certain country resources." In essence, "public health" would serve as a Trojan Horse to demolish national sovereignty and to transfer control of assets and the population to a global dictatorship.

The lure of technology is convenience. Convenience has blinded people to the danger of Digital IDs—which are designed to serve as weapons for centralized control. Digital IDs facilitate the transfer, sharing, and misuse of personal information by stealth financial and government agencies. Digital IDs are designed to block what the government declares to be unauthorized activities. Furthermore, digital IDs are twenty-four-hour surveillance weapons from which there is no escape. Digital IDs would facilitate digitally monitored concentration camps.

As has been noted by James Roguski, the proposed IHR amendments reveal that the "powers that be" are intent on "normalizing" the implementation of a global digital health certificate. He has compiled a list of the top 10 reasons to oppose the IHR amendments. These include:

- Changing the WHO "from an advisory organization ... to a governing body whose proclamations would be legally binding." (Articles 1 and 42)
- Removing language preserving "respect for dignity, human rights and fundamental freedoms of people." (Article 3)
- Giving the WHO "authority to require medical examinations, proof of prophylaxis, proof of vaccine and to implement contact tracing, quarantine and treatment." (Article 18)

- Instituting "a system of global health certificates in digital or paper format" (multiple articles and annexes)
- Empowering the WHO's Emergency Committee "to override decisions made by sovereign nations regarding health measures." (Article 43)

As Dr. Stoller notes, "tyranny runs on fear ... Tyranny can only be imposed if the population believes they are nothing more than their animal bodies limited to their five senses ... Tyranny cannot exist where there is freedom of speech. [It is] rather sad that the megalomanic leading this [diabolical plot] was again a German national, Klaus Schwab. One would have thought we were done with that part of our history."

# Introduction to the Revised Edition

Pharmakeia: a false hope and deception of false peace, false healing, and a false future.

This book is a revised edition of *Incurable Me* originally published by Skyhorse in 2016. Most books on medical practice will be completely outdated after five years, but the vast majority of *Incurable Me* remained relevant well beyond what should have been its expiration date.

As I write this new introduction to the first paperback edition of *Incurable Me*, now *Incurable Us*, we are still in the midst of the greatest worldwide psychological operation in the history of man. Not that long ago we were hunter-gatherers where family, purpose, cooperation, and community where paramount to survival. We were never wired to withstand the level of psychological manipulation we have been experiencing, the purpose of which was to invert reality so we could easily be led to slaughter. It has split our realities, and now we have two separate realities co-existing in the same space-time. The splitting of these two realities is inevitable: the only question is how will it happen (one funeral at a time, for example), and which one are you in?

As you will read in the original introduction, I showed how it takes about two years for citizens in the United States to recognize they are being poisoned and for our captured regulatory agencies to make some token, inadequate attempt to fix the problem. COVID demonstrated that it can take longer than two years for many to realize they and their families were subjected to an actual democide.

It started slowly; it started a century ago when the Rockefeller Foundation took over the practice of medicine. Then one-by-one Federal agencies developed mercantile relationships with the very companies they were supposed to be regulating—kind of an economic Stockholm Syndrome with Big Pharma. Pharma cares about one thing—profits—yet we have let this psychopathic entity run policy in multiple countries.

Big Pharma and the Department of Defense (CIA, etc.) worked hand–in–hand, to implement a control grid where everyone seemed to be taking orders from a central source … "Operation Lockstep" if you will … even though the population was kept in the dark. After all, you just don't announce there has been a Bio-Military-Security State coup of the US government (along with many other countries) and expect the population will be OK with that. When it came to COVID, the Federal Drug Administration (FDA) was MIA, the Centers for Disease Control and Prevention (CDC) was but rubberstamping because on a practical level there was no more CDC—they became the propaganda arm of Pharma prevaricating their dark little hearts out to the public. The FDA existed in name only when it came to COVID … it was all a military operation, perhaps in cooperation with China's Fifth Column war to take down the United States. The CDC actually had the public relations firm for Pfizer/Moderna embed themselves inside the CDC. The CDC is a regulatory agency; it is not supposed to be marketing the very things they are supposed to be regulating. But then they have been doing just that for all vaccines for decades and few complained. You never have the same entity in charge of promoting and distributing (that also owns patents) vaccines also be in charge of safety—that is a recipe for disaster.

It was an out-in-the-open fact that the National Institutes of Health (NIH) was funding Gain-of-Function research at the Wuhan lab.[1] In 2015, a paper was published, "A SARS -like cluster of circulation bat coronaviruses shows potential for human emergence." This study clearly states that the authors conducted Gain-of-Function research on bat coronaviruses in order to make them infectious to primary human airway epithelial cells. Ralph Baric and colleague Zhengli Shi were very much engineering the CoV2 virus in Wuhan to make sure that virus was highly infectious to humans. So, literally everything that came out of National Institute of Allergy and Infectious Diseases (NIAID) director Anthony Fauci's mouth and the rest of the government was gas-lighting.

## YE SHALL KNOW THEM BY THEIR FRUITS.

Western Civilization was targeted for destruction and subjected to an intense propaganda campaign to create a permanent global government, but beneath the psyop was this Fifth Column war against the United States and beneath that a spiritual war. Not being tangential here, but one can't ignore these macro disease issues—the spiritual sickness component of all this—and expect to understand the micro disease issues, such as how does one end one's addiction or bowel disease. Part of this spiritual war is to destroy the experiment called the United States—a Constitutional Republic where rights were given by God. That doesn't work for the imperialistic New World Order group. The United States was always the thorn in their side and had to be destroyed, and they got very far along in doing so—too far it seems. Bill Gates and Mark Zuckerberg have poured millions upon millions of dollars into the public education system in the United States, but students have only been getting dumber and dumber, so one has to assume all that money was not to improve education but to destroy it. You don't want your future slaves to be educated—indoctrinated, absolutely, but not educated. The dumbing down of Americans has been a goal of Skull & Bones for some time. Secret societies, like Skull & Bones, the Council of Foreign relations (CFR) (which is not so secret), Club of Rome, Committee of 300, etc., don't just want the destruction of the United States as a sovereign nation but want to destroy the ideals behind it. Ultimately, the goal is to deconstruct Christianity as well. These organizations are the domain of the highest-level puppets.

Nature, the creative spark of life, is an anathema to these groups of misanthropes who pretend they care about the environment. We are just useless eaters and bottom-feeders to them to be exploited and killed. I wish this was some bad science-fiction story, but there is actually a death cult that want to live the high-life on our corpses, and while they have many names, they are all as doomed as their plans. There is no reasoning with them—they will never figure it out—but we need to figure it out to end this. If we don't face this head-on, then Pharma will take over the world and will make sure, for example, that you can't travel if you are over fourteen and not taking a statin drug (assuming you have not already been culled).

Millions were being encouraged to illegally come to the United States and bring one of the bio-weapons being used to destroy us from the inside. Not CoV2, but fentanyl. Because the press, the legacy press, was captured and carried water for these enemies and traitors, the failsafe that would have prevented all this was removed. Without the media, CoV2 would have just been another flu-like illness that primarily affected the elderly and those with multiple co-morbidities. Overall mortality did not go up in 2020, but it did in 2021 when the death jab was rolled out. Remember how the flu completely disappeared in 2020? The media truly was the virus and also made sure you didn't know the United States was being invaded by design.

Well, the flu never disappeared. It was just called COVID to juice the numbers in a casedemic extraordinaire. We actually saw our hospitals become de facto euthanasia factories, inappropriately putting patients on ventilators and pumping them full of the deadly drug Remdesivir (what nurses called "Run-Your-Death-is Near"). I always wondered if all the videos of dancing nurses were their way of telling the public that hospitals were not being overwhelmed with COVID patients. But there was no science supporting the use of Remdesivir, and it was known as a deadly drug that was killing Ebola victims in a drug trial so its use was halted. But the regulatory gatekeepers were all compromised, fired, or had resigned in disgust. The hospitals received a 20 percent payment bonus if they used the drug. A $500,000 hospital bill would generate an extra $150,000 if Remdesivir was used. Putting a patient on a ventilator earned the hospital $40,000. A lot of money to help hospitals make choices about priorities (wink, wink).

Media organizations played a central role, especially Big Tech IT companies, in stifling anything that wasn't the approved narrative. Mainstream scientists, many leading experts in their field, working in prestigious institutions, and some medical journal editors themselves were all silenced, while others were paid off. Where were all the billions coming from to create fabricated research critical of effective early interventions such as hydroxychloroquine (HCQ) and Ivermectin? How much did the *New England Journal of Medicine* and *The Lancet* get from FTX (the criminal crypto group) to publish articles so obviously flawed they would have been the cause of expulsion from any academic center that still had any integrity? FTX was critical in funding the attacks on effective early interventions with the resultant loss of life.

FTX founder Sam Bankman-Fried had Wall Street and the media in his pocket while he practiced effective altruism (a.k.a. deceit that makes one look like a moral leader). But it was just another Ponzi scheme that was funding favorite New World Order players. It happened right out in the open. Bankman-Fried's mother was apparently responsible for running major voter harvesting operations in the 2020 election, so the FTX group was a critical component of a fraudulent government and its fraudulent economy.

Wonder why it was so important to keep the conflict in Ukraine going while sabotaging efforts at peace negotiations? Yeah, it was a money laundering operation, and they never wanted it to end, even if the end was an all-out nuclear holocaust. Few knew Ukraine was the playground for the dark ones—the local population didn't know any more than US citizens knew their country is actually the headquarters of the dark ones and that our Constitutional Republic vanished years ago. Drug trafficking, sex trade, organ harvesting, etc. were all taking place in Ukraine without any interference until the Russian invasion.

## PANDEMIC/SCAMDEMIC

A century of pandemic preparedness protocols were trashed so a psychotic, pipsqueak, criminal mastermind could enrich himself and his loyal following (loyal because he controlled their NIH grants). We were literally in the middle of a *Godfather* movie, but it wasn't Don Corleone calling the shots: It was dog torturer, vivisectionist extraordinaire, Don "I am the Science" Fauci. There was some truth to that statement, though, because this one man literally was the point man for distributing tens of billions of dollars to academic and research institutions throughout the world, so he had almost complete control of the "science." This was a very dark, pernicious situation; for example, if a research team finds out that it is very dangerous to inject vaccines that contain aluminum (80 percent of vaccines contain aluminum), that research team will be defunded and journals will be told not to print their research papers.

Eighty-six percent of the world was shut down for an infection that had a 0.035 percent mortality from zero to fifty-nine years of age and 0.095 percent mortality for the post-sixty set.[2] If you were younger than twenty, the fatality rate was 0.0003 percent. Clearly, this is below fatality rates from the flu, and yet this was the emergency that allowed them to bypass safety studies and force/coerce people to get experimental injections that had never been used before and lie about what they would do. They lied when saying the "vaccine" would prevent transmission and infection and that it was, of course, safe and effective, as they say all vaccines are … safe and effective became an indoctrination mantra. Vaccines do not have adequate safety studies despite what we have all been led to believe. This was not just regulatory maleficence—this was about trashing the US Constitution and murdering as many as possible in the process. An inconvenient truth to be sure, but the masses are slow to acknowledge that their own governments and the medical profession would deliberately murder their fellows—a regrettable but predictable outcome of our unlovely, amoral society. The main mission of the World Health Organiszation (WHO) is population control—not a lot of us know that.

As I write this, the median/mean age of death from COVID holds steady at eighty-two years of age. Seventy percent of the mortalities in the United States were in the elderly with six or more underlying medical conditions. If it were not going to be COVID, it would have been something else as they were already beyond the average life expectancy. Over the last three years, no healthy child in the United States died from a CoV2 infection … not a single healthy child.

Meanwhile, a New Zealand Ministry of Health database administrator-turn-whistleblower showed that certain batches of the COVID jab were killing as many as 21 percent of those receiving the jab (December 2023). This wasn't just in New Zealand but increases in mortality were taking place all over the world (that had received the death jab, because not all countries pushed it, especially not in Africa).

We weren't supposed to be alive to discuss any of this, but the criminal "reset" plan failed out of the starting gate because it was the hope of the Globalists that CoV2 would have killed billions, and the jab was just supposed to finish off as many survivors as possible. Too many people were left alive asking inconvenient questions. One of the few true responsibilities of a government is to protect its citizens and the integrity of the nation's border, but the so-called "open border" was intended to bring in a replacement population, because the rest of us were supposed to be already dead or dying, but what a great way to justify bringing in a digital ID and to track your carbon footprint—also important to keep track of millions of military-age men from China to Zaire (Democratic Republic of the Congo). By the way, the carbon they want to get rid of is us.

## IF YOU CAN'T DEFINE THE ENEMY YOU CAN'T DEFEAT YOUR ENEMY

So, please indulge me as I explain this attempt at planetary genocide. One of the things that makes fleshing out these events important is medicine as we have known it will not survive—the population is losing and will soon lose completely any trust in public health institutions and modern medicine in general, and that trust won't be coming back any time soon nor should it. Evidence Based Medicine (EBM) was destroyed during the last few years and public health decisions were being made on plausibility, as in how much money is it plausible to make if we force deadly injections on the public that don't even work and lock them down?

Modern medicine decided to follow a dark agenda and became a dark influence. While COVID may have been a Hail Mary for the dying paradigm of the Bio-Military-Pharmaceutical complex to maintain control, it still caused a lot of death and suffering. The lockdown fetishism imposed on us was an import from China, but it was also the agenda of the New World Order (NWO)/World Economic Forum (WEF) set.

Human history has been replete with invasions, attacks, trade wars, etc. It seems like raging war on each other was chosen to be the primary operational paradigm on this planet. For the most part people were driven by the need to eat, have land to grow food and to establish trade routes, etc. I am not assigning blame; after all, it was the crucible of our modern civilization, which I have to say has not turned out so well. Today, war is a machine—unending and on anything and everything, be it COVID, drugs, terrorism, Afghanistan, Ukraine, the Mid-East—it doesn't matter. The population is never told the real reasons for war, which is to wash money out of our hands and into the hands of this group of dark elites. So, war is never over; there is always another, and it never stops.

Energetically, Earth was being beset upon by a dark energy that was not home grown; it was only present because there were enough humans who held the negative traits necessary for this energy to become interested in feeding off of them and the havoc they could reap. The generation of fear is key to its survival or presence on this planet—fear (the opposite of love) is the gasoline this dark force runs on.

But what does any of this esoterica have to do with the US government, the largest empire in modern times—an empire that became vicious, incompetent, utterly corrupt, and under the control of agendas pushed from elsewhere? This immigrant invasion had only one purpose once it was clear millions didn't die from COVID—to destroy the United States and other Western countries from within.

> "We know that they are lying, they know that they are lying, they even know that we know they are lying, we also know that they know we know they are lying too, they of course know that we certainly know they know we know they are lying too as well, but they are still lying. In our country, the lie has become not just moral category, but the pillar industry of this country."
>
> — Aleksandr Solzhenitsyn

Since it seems politicians lie and can't stop themselves from lying, the public lost the ability to know big lies from small lies—call it some kind of desensitization but it produced an apathy that only empowered the cabal. Institutionalized lying is a major factor that enables liars-in-chief to carry out their illegal, immoral, and criminal practices of institutionalized discrimination, retaliation, defamation, and intellectual harassment.

Deception is the modus operandi of the dark ones, which is why free speech had to be eliminated in their playbook. Puppets are never told the true reasons for doing what they are doing, only the upper tier of puppets are made privy to some of this information. For example, the CIA hitman who murdered Marylin Monroe was told she was sleeping with Fidel Castro and leaking to him things JFK had whispered to her under the sheets (she was not sleeping with Castro, but typically the dark ones lie to their puppets). Normand Hodges said he carried out thirty-seven assassinations for the United States between 1959–1972.

Jumping ahead in this story to address one of the top puppets, Peter Daszak, who is a perfect example of how this dark energy turns the like-minded into its puppets. Can you believe that a scientist funded by the US government could possibly create a virus on purpose to release it and then hype up a resulting infectious disease crisis all for profit and power?

> Daszak reiterated that, until an infectious disease crisis is very real, present, and at an emergency threshold, it is often largely ignored. To sustain the funding base beyond the crisis, he said, we need to increase public understanding of the need for MCMs (medical countermeasures) such as a pan-influenza or pan-coronavirus vaccine. A key driver is the media, and the economics follow the hype. We need to use that hype to our advantage to get to the real issues. Investors will respond if they see profit at the end of process, Daszak stated.

The previous paragraph is from page 73 of "Rapid Medical Countermeasure Response to Infectious Diseases: Enabling Sustainable Capabilities Through Ongoing Public and Private-Sector Partnerships"—published by the National Academy of Sciences in 2016.[3]

We know so little about the true history of mankind on this planet—the great civilizations that have waxed and waned long before recorded modern history.[4] Regardless of the time or place, oligarchs of the civilizations that we do know about have been obsessed with over-population going back to at least the days of Plato (Plato [De republica, V] and Aristotle [De republica, II, vi]). While, there are some areas on the planet that have too many humans in the same space or in the wrong place, over-population itself is a myth perpetuated to help the ruling class maintain control—it is about wealth transfer. Even though most of humanity is not aware of the full extent of what has been going on, open war has been declared by those who want to repress and command with the purpose of keeping the rest of us unconscious, keeping us from being inquiring beings, and keeping us from knowing how strong the human spirit is or exploring what we are capable of becoming. This is the emotional grid they want to impose. They want to keep us small and controlled so they can feed off of our assets and energies. They are literally deranged fools whose minds have been warped by their greed and the covenant they have made with forces that have always lied to them and continue to lie to them. This struggle is not new and is addressed in fable and parable by many of the world's ancient texts, but this is not speculation of what has happened in the far past—this is about what is happening now and why.

*Lose your Spirit and you have lost everything ... Lionel Richie (singer/songwriter)*

It is problematic that humans think they are nothing more than evolved mammalian primates (apes). Yes, those are the bodies we use, but we are spiritual beings having a human experience, not just naked apes that aspire to be spiritual. Spirit is not the enthusiasm you have for your local high school football team. It would behoove us all to try and understand what spirit is because there have been those trying to kill you for having one. There are energies and powers connected with being human—a subject about which humans are almost completely unaware; however, there are those who know about these hidden features of the human experience and want those energies and powers for themselves. Without belaboring the point, tyranny can only be imposed if the population believes they are nothing more than their animal bodies limited to their five senses. Tyranny runs on fear, and it is much harder to scare someone who is not completely tied to what their five senses tell them reality is all about. Tyranny cannot exist where there is freedom of speech so it is really easy to tell who the "bad" guys are … they censor and don't want freedom of speech.

## WHERE THIS TIMELINE STARTS

In a timeline that starts in 1933, although the darkness got its foothold long before that, a group of bankers hatched a plot to replace US President Franklin D. Roosevelt with someone who was more in line with these entrenched institutions and the systemic ideologies that do not want democracies to exist. These dark ones were still drunk on their success from being able to create the Federal Reserve. There was no coup d'état because their point man, retired Marine Corps General Smedley Butler, betrayed them. So, the banking cabal shifted all their attention to Germany.

That same year the Public Health Service of the United States began its infamous Tuskegee Experiment on poor black males in Alabama. An experiment that lasted forty years and only ended in 1972 because of a leak to the press. Under the guise of receiving free health care, the victims were watched to see what the ravages of syphilis would do to them and their families. No Nuremberg trial held, no accountability—but if you are an American, apparently, it's okay to say you were just following orders if caught, and it's all *mea culpa* and asking for amnesty.

The lessons of the last century have not been completely understood, and now humanity is in that awkward place where there is a reckoning with these poorly understood experiences that have been swept under the rug. However, the rug is now gone and it would behoove the world to recognize the players of our immediate past for who they really were. For example, Adolf Hitler was probably the greatest teacher of hate the twentieth century had ever seen. Intolerance was intense in the western world a century ago, and he filled the role others had prepared for someone with this intention and influence. He had other options for his life, which he closed down early.

Yes, I know once you bring up Hitler or suggest we are unduly influenced by energies we can't perceive many will just tune out, but that is merely a reflection of how indoctrinated we have all become. Indoctrinated by negative energies that have kept us trapped for millennia in deception, delusion, fear, and wars, and part of that indoctrination was to convince us we were powerless to change any of this. Rather sad that the megalomaniac leading this for WEF was again a German national, Klaus Schwab. One would have thought we were done with that part of our history.

This is what WWII was about ... Hitler, like Schwab, was merely a tool for large international corporations and banks that were funding him to implement a top-down feudal economy in Europe that would hopefully expand worldwide and reign for a thousand years or as long as they had the slaves to feed into the system. Yet, their tool became too unstable, too unpredictable, and too uncontrollable as he tried to take over the entire planet. The globalists were still able to use him as a pretext for the NATO/European Union (EU) paradigm to control Europe. Now, with both the inspiration for Hitler and much of his financial support coming from inside the United States, it was no surprise that Operation Paperclip brought so many Nazi scientists and technocrats to the United States after the kinetic war was completed (approximately 30,000 Nazis). The American Nazis—although, they did not call themselves Nazis—brought their assets back while Hitler himself, a deletant compared to the fools who have made war against us today, was allowed to retire to South America.[5]

The eugenicists in America were a great influence and inspiration to the Nazi regime and, in fact, the movement was a part of the defense used in the Nuremberg trials to justify the programs the Nazis implemented. But there were other influencers, as well, and they may still be present today. The upper tier of Nazidom was deeply into the dark side of occult esoterica. The swastika itself is an ancient symbol of the universe so what the Nazis did was use that symbol rotated to the left or counter-clockwise—a symbol of a devolving universe, not an evolving universe shown when it rotates to the right.[6]

This symbol drew in those worldwide who knew what it meant (rotating counter clockwise), which is why, for example, dead Tibetans were reported to have been found among the casualties in WWII ... sorcerers perhaps enlisted to help with dark rituals. Rituals are really important to the puppets of darkness as it provides them with a sense of power. They are now flaunting some of their rituals in the open; just to name three—the weird closing Olympic ceremony in London 2012, which heralded a plague that would put many in hospital.[7] In late 2021, the rapper Travis Scott's Astroworld performance was not only overtly satanic but murders (human sacrifices?) took place during the performance.[8] In 2022, there were also the overtly satanic advertisements of Balenciaga.[9]

It would surprise many to find out just who these puppets of darkness have been and currently are. For example, Madeleine Albright, former secretary of state, was celebrated when she passed in 2022, despite being a mass murderer. She publicly announced that the sanctions that were imposed on Iraq that killed over half a million children were worth it. Research who has attended the ceremonies at Bohemian Grove (Northern California) where they worship the false deity Molech, and you may be surprised.[10] Then there is the Bilderberg/Davos group and their High Priests (that is literally what they call themselves)—a smarmier group of international corporate scum and villainy you will never find. The World Economic Forum (WEF) is just a front group for these power crazed psychopaths who draw into their circle those who are in synch with them (the Law of Attraction).

Consider the possibility that we are part of a universe replete with life and intelligence of all types and stripes, be they seen or unseen—trillions upon trillions of conscious beings to a greater or lesser degree. It is regrettable that humans are so unaware and so misinformed about our participation in the cosmos, and we are even less aware of non-humans in the affairs of our lives and our planet. Some seem to be divinely angelic; some are more like predatory parasites. The point being, like attracts-like regardless of whether one is human, a bird, a fish or an interdimensional being.

As questionable as the influence of these low vibrational "others" might be, they probably weren't responsible for the descent of certain governments into satanic, murderous, pedophilic networks used to control and manipulate those that entered the halls of power. Pedophilia is the sick glue that holds their system together. The dark ones know children, especially young children, are closer to Source and by defiling them, by being brutal and cruel, one is showing God that you are a counterion—an angry counterion. Why would you want to show God you are an angry counterion? Seems counter-intuitive, but foolish humans believed the promises made to them about personal power and wealth, so for the weak minded ... that apparently is all it takes, as unfortunately there are many with weak minds.

This is beyond mere corruption; world governments had been bled out from the inside by these global predators. In fact, international banks, working with Pfizer, successfully executed a planetary coup against the nation-state. Pfizer is the most criminally fined corporation in America that admitted in front of the European Union that they never tested the COVID injection to see if it would stop transmission or infection. Of course, now we know it doesn't.

One of the predators, who actually was and may never have stopped being a Nazi is global financier and convicted felon George Soros.[11] His plan, which is shared by many in these elite circles, was to shut down every part of the economy in the first world, and de-industrialize the United States. The collapsing borders, super-inflation, total elimination of fossil fuels (unless it comes from perhaps British Petroleum or Saudi Arabia because they seem to be in league with the globalists), and collapse of the world food supply (mass starvation) were all created so a corporate UN-coordinated world government can come in and act as saviors and impose their anti-terraforming religion where carbon dioxide will be removed from the atmosphere in the name of being Green. Green was intended to be the new anti-human, anti-science religion used to isolate, control, and eventually eliminate as much as 80 percent of the human population on the planet, for the carbon they really want to remove is us. If Green were really "Green," why are we outsourcing our energy needs to China where slaves are many and human rights are few? Those batteries for electric cars require cobalt mined by exploited African children. Who do you think is making all those Chinese solar panels (yes, they make most of them)? How about a million Uyghur Muslim slaves incarcerated because of their religion —at least until someone with money needs an organ that matches one of the slaves, be they Muslim or Falun Gong practitioners. It's called Green Washing, or environmental virtue signaling.

A massive global death cult has been lurking for decades for the moment to strike. They actually believed they could transcend carbon-based life and have their consciousness transferred to some silicon-based life-form. In the short term, their plan is to neutralize the United States with a civil war/economic collapse while China takes over the South China Sea including Taiwan.

Whether you personally believe in malevolence, Satan,[12] or nasty inter-dimensionals is your choice, but the globalists believe in them and most have sold their proverbial souls[13] for something they already had, and now they have created a covenant with the losing team. The weird thing is on some level they know it, but can't stop themselves, so they push forward with their deranged game plans to create a transhuman world where most humans have been eliminated, and they want this all to happen by 2030 according to their own published agenda.[14]

A world that will be free of poverty and hunger because we won't be in it, but those who remain will own nothing, be happy, and eat bugs—again, this plan has been cooking for the last century. The globalists' desire to be top dogs on a prison planet is so intense their wish may actually be granted, but not on this Earth. That seems to be the way a benevolent universe works; you get what you want, eventually, but it may not be exactly how you planned it out. Be that as it may, there also seems to be a lot of malevolence tolerated at certain levels and layers of our reality, undoubtedly to stir the evolutionary pot for the benefit of all. Nevertheless, what goes around comes around, so if true, you don't trade your future for temporary misuse of power, as seductive as it may be. It is a poor choice, but some insist on learning the hard way, yet even in their insanity, the lessons they offer benefit the whole.

## MEDICAL TYRANNY AND SOFT KILL WEAPONS

Fluoride seems to have been the first foray into medical tyranny to control populations. The historical use of fluoride for behavior control probably started in the

Soviet gulags in the 1930s, but Nazi Germany was quick to apply the same in their prison camps as the mineral makes humans apathetic and easy to dominate—stupid and docile. The propaganda campaign in the United States was so convincing that fluoride was essential for preventing tooth decay that anyone who questioned its use in the water supply, even though fluoride is more poisonous than lead, was considered a nut case. The book *The Fluoride Deception* is well-researched and goes over this in detail.[15]

The practice and paradigm of fluoridating municipal drinking water demonstrated that the public would accept drinking poison if the government insisted it was a public health measure being done for the benefit of citizen's well-being—*"Fur Ihre Sicherheit"* or "it's for your safety," a common Nazi refrain. This poison is still universally defended by the dentists who will willingly put the most poisonous non-radioactive element on the periodic table in your mouth, mercury amalgam fillings, and call it silver. The mercury is constantly leeching out and you breathe it in and swallow it too.

During WWII, the biowarfare activities of the Japanese were particularly atrocious. As many as three thousand allied troops lost their lives in places such as the infamous Unit 731 testing biologics, as well as an untold number of civilians when these agents were released in Asia. The United States covertly granted the scientists involved immunity not unlike Operation Paper Clip.[16]

Blame it on the fluoridated water, but we have allowed ourselves to be experimented on far too easily and without holding anyone accountable. There is no freedom without accountability. In 1950, the US Army sprayed the bacteria serratia marcescens in San Francisco from a boat(s) in the bay—Operation Sea Spray—and continued until 1969. There was at least one documented death from the infections that followed.

Infantile paralysis or polio didn't exist until the heavy use of various pesticides, the most notable being DDT, which is required to weaken the immune system so a previously benign stomach virus could start causing paralysis. But the government had encouraged and required the liberal use of DDT, and it was used everywhere and on almost everything (still is in certain parts of the world). Nevertheless, a virus and only a virus would be blamed for what was actually an illness caused by a pesticide, or else there would be great liability to both the government and industry. So fear of a virus was ginned up—sound familiar? The mass vaccination campaign initially gave millions a retrovirus infection, a simian virus (SV40), now known to be causally related to several types of cancer.

Don't misunderstand what is written here ... an enterovirus causes the illness but it needs a toxic co-factor in most cases. If the truth of the toxic cause of polio was known, and the government held accountable for infecting millions with a cancer-causing retrovirus, we would not be where we are today. The first mass vaccination program for polio in the United States, now called the Cutter Incident, gave 200,000 children polio. To convince the public the polio vaccine program was working, the definition of polio was changed so that one had to be paralyzed for at least sixty days to be classified as having polio—most cases resolved before sixty days, and of course they knew that. It made the vaccine look very effective. Today, the definition of what is a vaccine has been redefined to accommodate a hard-to-sell, problematic gene-transfer therapy that makes the human body create a pathogenic protein, potentially sterilizes[17] many recipients, and inflames their hearts.[18] Make the human body produce a pathogenic spike protein—what could go wrong?

Oh, and the definition of "Gain-of-Function" was changed as well, so the reader can decide if that made Dr. Fauci look any more credible. Especially when it was found he wanted EcoHealth Alliance to spray more virulent coronavirus in Wuhan caves to infect the local population (the Pentagon refused to fund the project—maybe because it was an act of war?).[19]

## MADE IN THE USA

By masking biowarfare programs as public health measures producing vaccines, these fools were able to get around restrictions. The Department of Defense (DOD) and Defense Advanced Research Projects Agency (DARPA) admitted to operating forty-six biolabs in Ukraine, for public health of course, but pay no attention to the fact we operate these labs all over the world … "we are the good guys." In 2012, DARPA developed their ADEPT:PROTECT project that would use gene-encoded vaccines to stop a pandemic (that they would then create?). There was no WARP speed program—Pfizer had the first patent on a coronavirus vaccine in 1990 long before Trump announced WARP speed. And they found out it didn't work because coronavirus mutates so fast and so often that it is not a candidate for vaccines. There have now been thousands of published research articles saying it does not work, so if you want to "follow the science" it was there all along for many years, and this science has never been disputed.

Moderna got its first contract in 2013[20], but it was the DOD that came up with the idea of mRNA vaccines—this whole thing has been a military operation from the get go. By 2015, the peer-reviewed literature had articles announcing the enhanced CoV2 was ready to be used (on the human population). It was never a China-virus; the Wuhan lab was just enhancing what was created in the United States. Within the first week thousands of pregnant women were taking this vaccine. Never have we given experimental vaccines to pregnant women. In the past, medicine went out of its way to protect pregnant women from as much as possible, certainly including interventions that would upset their immune systems, but medicine was now neutered—only Pharmakeia existed and was in full control.

The polio outbreak showed that you could herd the sheep (humans in this case) into a slaughter house if there was an invisible enemy; a virus is perfect for that because one can use fear to get populations to turn to their government to protect them from this invisible enemy. If you have control of the media, you can also implement a divide and conquer strategy, so if you can turn men against women, blacks against whites, heterosexuals against LGBTQ+ people, established populations against immigrants—all of that causes people to turn to their governments for interventions. Do you think those funding Critical Race Theory and Drag Queen Story-Time want harmony? No, they want culture wars.

In the United States, if one disagreed with the narrative of the media, the Department of Justice or FBI would label that individual either a domestic terrorist or white supremacist/racist regardless of their skin color. It was part of the plan to blame the destruction of the United States on white supremacists, but ponder this one example—the City of Oakland, California is deeply beset with crime and violence, but I would challenge you to find even one white supremist in Oakland. Those behind the tyrannical cult we have been subjected to are not super-intelligent, but few realize they get their power from public acquiescence and those whose perceptions they have to control. Yes, the cult has a lot of financial resources and many deluded minions who will blindly do their bidding, but they are weak—only the weak censor. The censorship was a desperate move to control perceptions. But the censorship surrounding COVID killed tens of thousands.

So, with a virus, you can stop people from gathering, organizing, and if you can digitize a population, you can control who is talking to whom and where. If you can get people to attend school online or do their work online from home, the government can listen to everything everyone is saying and writing and buying. The excuse is that it is *"Fur Ihre Sicherheit"* to protect against the invisible enemy. It also keeps people lonely, isolated, and depressed. People will buy into solutions before they know anything about the consequences of that solution, so you can mandate lockdowns without proper science supporting them, injections that have not been adequately tested, or vaccines that are known to cause harm for the greater good of someone's bottom-line.

## INFECTIOUS DISEASE SKULLDUGGERY

This is not a comprehensive tome of infectious disease skullduggery, but in 1955 it was reported that the CIA conducted an open-air biological warfare experiment near Tampa, Florida and environs with the Pertussis bacteria. It was alleged that the nasty endeavor tripled the whooping cough infections in Florida to over one-thousand cases and caused whooping cough deaths in the state to increase twelve-fold over the previous year.[21]

In 1966, the US Army released Bacillus globigii into the tunnels of the New York City Subway system, as part of a field experiment called "A Study of the Vulnerability of Subway Passengers in New York City to Covert Attack with Biological Agents." The Chicago subway system was also subject to a similar experiment by the Army.[22]

Bacillus globigii was used to simulate an attack with anthrax, but as it turned out, now we know this bacterium is a human pathogen.[23]

The US government conducted many radiation experiments on the unwary, MKULTRA drug experiments on the unknowing, and torture experiments on the incarcerated, but again … this is not meant to be a comprehensive list. By the time US President Eisenhower left office with his infamous speech warning us to beware the "military-industrial-complex," we were being lead into unending military conflicts, often initiated by false flag events such as the Gulf of Tonkin incident that was used to start the Vietnam War.

## MEN IN BLACK

In the 1950s, the CIA had split into two factions. The western faction was almost exclusively in control of anything that had to do with extraterrestrials—I don't mention this to be sensational. In the years that followed, the military-industrial paradigm evolved and became inclusive of many multinational corporations, investment houses, and banks, which benefited from this arrangement and led to the current massive corporate interests, such as Black Rock/Vanguard, which span the globe and whose shareholder-ships are networked among a very small oligarch class.

While President Roosevelt avoided a coup, President John F. Kennedy did not, and he was assassinated (1963) in a coordinated plot managed by the CIA's E. Howard Hunt. Lyndon B. Johnson was vice president and was fully aware of the planned elimination of JFK, as was the infamous director of the FBI, J. Edgar Hoover. Apparently, America decided to explore the dark side and so begin unending wars and skullduggery around the globe. But I doubt this could have been possible without the cooperation of the press in covering up the facts of the event. Why was Kennedy assassinated?

Kennedy wanted the United States back on the gold standard, he wanted the CIA dismantled, and he never wanted the United States to get entangled in Vietnam. Unbeknownst to Kennedy, the CIA had become far more than the "CIA"; they were literally the Men in Black in matters extraterrestrial, and if the CIA was threatened it also threatened the cover being used in such matters and the monopoly of information the CIA had on this information. Kennedy had a vision for the space program, but his vison was not shared by those using NASA as a front organization for their secret space program (they were back engineering crashed vehicles, probably with the help of low-vibrational ETs, but that is speculation).[24] Just days before his murder, Kennedy signed an agreement with Kurschev to cooperate on moon exploration and signed an executive order requesting the CIA share what they knew about UFOs to make sure there were no accidents from confusing UFOs with an aggressive act by either side. The CIA had no intention of sharing anything with anyone and certainly wasn't going to let the chief executive tell them what to do even if that meant making him "wet," as in sleeping with the fishes.

Meanwhile, the secret biowarfare facility located on Plum Island off the coast of Connecticut was developing an enhanced version of the Borrelia bacteria (Lyme disease) under the directorship of former German SS-officer and microbiologist Eric Traub—Gain-of-Function research. This organism with increased virulence now infects 20 percent of the world's population. Be that as it may, the virulence of the organism was not robust enough for the globalists.

The fall-guy set-up to take the blame for the JFK assassination was CIA asset Lee Harvey Oswald, who strangely enough was reported to be mixed up in a virus gain-of-function program for the purpose of developing a weapon that would kill Fidel Castro. Oswald knew too much and was expendable, so he was a convenient "patsy." Mary Sherman, the scientist running the program, was murdered. It is still speculation whether there was a link to this apparent effort to create a deadly virus and the subsequent identification and possible enhancement of the HIV virus.

Maurice Hillerman, one of the world's most prominent virologists of his time and a vice president of Merck, was recorded boasting, "So we brought African Greens in and I didn't know we were importing the AIDS virus at the time."[25] Merck switched from Indian rhesus to green monkeys because the rhesus monkeys were full of retroviruses including SV40. Was HIV just due to sloppy virology, or was HIV, once identified, manipulated and chosen as a bioweapon? A weapon that must have been a big disappointment as it took far too long to kill its victims. Intentional or not, in all likelihood it was introduced in the United States via the Hepatitis B vaccine trials that exclusively recruited gay men in New York, San Francisco, and Los Angeles. The bottom-line is that vaccineologists in the twentieth century were creating invasive medical interventions with no clue as to what they were doing and as a result murdered many. Or did they know what they were doing?

The situation in Africa is a little less clear; starting in 1957,[26] oral polio vaccines were administered by the Wistar Institute and given to "hundreds of thousands of Africans." As with almost all vaccines, there was no follow-up. The FDA has archived vaccines from that period, and if they forensically looked at them to see if HIV was present, they have not told anyone. That would eliminate the conspiracy theories, but it would also implicate the whole vaccine program as a very problematic, unethical, and sloppy endeavor, to say the least.

Big Pharma, in the United States, was able to get unconditional liability protection from lawsuits related to adverse events from their vaccines in 1986. Safety was no longer their concern as the responsibility of vaccine safety was now the responsibility of the US government. So, there was an explosion of vaccines required for children and a mysterious increase in sudden infant death syndrome (SIDS), chronic health conditions, and a formerly rare neurological disorder called autism. Autism is a post-vaccination encephalitis but the connection between vaccines, mercury, aluminum (found in approximately 80 percent of vaccines at toxic levels), acetaminophen, and autism was deliberately covered up by agencies of the US government. When the CDC had the objective data that showed the vaccines were connected to autism, their response was to shred the data. A high-level whistleblower came forward and disclosed this, but no one in government did anything—no hearings, no investigation, nothing. This was the subject of the documentary *Vaxxed*.

Big Pharma was already well on its way to capturing regulatory agencies and politicians. No one in the upper echelons of government would dare reveal what they knew, and they never did; however, that silence empowered the eugenics cult. The US government never met their obligations under the National Childhood Vaccine Injury Act of 1986 and ignored all safety issues even as they pushed the mantra "Safe and Effective" so that by the time CoV2 showed up, the population was good and indoctrinated. Health and Human Services (HHS) already had decades of blowing off its statutory responsibilities for vaccine safety under its belt and few seemed to care.

SARS-1, the predecessor to SARS-2 (CoV2) arrived on the scene in 2002, and in all likelihood was a test run. The reason one does not here about it anymore is that is has no natural host, and therefore not in circulation. If there is no natural host, then where did it come from? Is there a wet market in the Wuhan virology lab? CoV2 was a made in the United States, but was sent to the Wuhan Virology Lab for enhancements that became illegal to do in the United States.

There is strong circumstantial evidence that A/H1N1, the so-called novel Mexican Swine flu event of 2009, was neither Mexican nor novel, but a genetically engineered creation from the United States. The virus included genetic bits of North American human, avian and swine flus, and Eurasian swine flu—the virus had not been detected in any pigs except those in a single herd in Canada.[27] A variant of A/H1N1 broke out in India in 2015, but has apparently not been a player since. No natural host.

Had there been a sincere and honest attempt to flesh out the origins of these viruses, again we would not be where we are today. While A/H1N1 was very infectious, the virus was no more problematic than the normal flu virus and has vanished. It may have just been a test run for a future release.

The attempt to scare the world with the Zika virus was a really big flop. They would not make that mistake again. The media was so quick to blame a relatively benign virus for the clusters of microcephaly in Brazil. However, too many found out fairly quickly that the pocket of mothers in Brazil who gave birth to children with microcephaly were vaccinated with DTP while pregnant and also drinking larvicide-laden tap water at the same time. So, that attempt to scare the world had to be shut down immediately because a vaccine was clearly implicated. At the same time a seminal paper was published—a retrospective look (using matched controls) at thirty years of DTP use in Africa showing an increased overall mortality ten-fold, so it was very important to shut down any interest in looking at the safety and efficacy of the DTP[28]

This brings us to CoV2 and the announcement by Dr. Anthony Fauci in 2017 that a surprise outbreak was imminent. The plot was apparently hatched as far back as 1999, at the University of North Carolina. In the subsequent years numerous white papers, such as SARS 2025-2028,[29] and the pandemic war games, such as Event 201,[30] were priming both the media and the public. Finally, they would have the event that would allow them to bring in their great reset of the world economy and cull the population at the same time. Key players in multiple governments had already been compromised, regulatory agencies had been captured, and Big Pharma, along with Big Tech, was in total control of conventional media outlets.

Yet, the CoV2 virus was not an infectious disease hellion. It took out the old and the infirm just like influenza does every year, so the hype had to go into overdrive, which the PCR tests accomplished—cycled so high clean swabs would test positive. It was critical that the number of deaths for CoV2 be very high in order to generate the fear to justify what would come next. So, despite long-standing rules for data collection and reporting, successfully used for years by all hospitals, medical examiners, coroners, and physicians. The overall mortality for 2020 did not increase from previous years, so the CDC changed the way they wanted deaths reported. Had they used the normal criteria, the mortality figures would have had to be revised down 90 percent. This is not to say the All-Cause-mortality didn't increase as it very much did in 2021 and 2022—New Zealand, which kept every good records, showed a 20 percent overall increase in mortality. Batch one of the COVID jabs caused a 21 percent mortality rate from the injection alone.

The very people within government who might have sounded the alarm that we were being manipulated into a bio-security state based on false information were compromised, as many of them would be able to earn millions of dollars from the licensing of the mRNA technology. It has been determined that almost half of all PCR results were false positives, which if nothing else calls into question the clinical trials used to validate the "vaccine."[31] As an aside, we have never had a vaccine that makes the human body create a pathogen in a controlled way for an uncontrolled duration. The spike protein is a significant pathogen—a loaded weapon if you will—with no assurance it would control the outbreak. We were lied to. It did not remain in the arm and nearby lymph nodes as we were told. The mRNA wasn't actually mRNA but a modified mRNA that the body could not easily breakdown. Spike proteins were being made, as per the instructions in the experimental jab, in the ovaries, the testes, the brain and the heart for undetermined time periods.

What happened next was fifty countries panicked and were cajoled into signing secret agreements with Pfizer, essentially putting them into receivership in exchange for the injections and monetary assistance from the World Bank and the International Monetary Fund.[32] The agreement was to remain secret for fifty years. Any criticism of the injections or of Pfizer would be forbidden, and Pfizer would not only direct the global response but also the response individual countries would have so a worldwide extermination system could be initiated. The FDA, now under operational control of the DOD, even asked a federal court to allow them fifty-five years to hold onto the data they relied on to give Emergency Use Authorization for the Pfizer injection. There can only be one reason for this request, and that is the FDA and DOD didn't want anyone to see that the Pfizer data showed that, at best, one would have to inject 22,000 people to potentially prevent one death. No need to point out the Wuhan A strain was no longer in circulation. I am also sure they didn't want anyone to see that there were more deaths in the injected group than in the control group.

The lack of early prevention and treatment protocols, and the persecution of anyone trying to treat COVID patients prior to hospitalization, was not a form of treatment nihilism; it was a well-organized, well-funded conspiracy to make sure nothing would interfere with an injection rollout. Never have sick patients been turned away from hospitals and told to come back when their lips were blue.

All the big players were deeply, corruptly, and maliciously in bed with Pharma, so would lose billions if it were found off-patent drugs could treat COVID. The FDA, under the direction of the DOD, illegally exercised emergency use powers and was a willing ally in the suppression of treatments known to be effective against the virus, such as something as benign as vitamin D. In some countries, physicians were arrested for prescribing ivermectin. Then injections were illegally marketed to children as well after the FDA advisory panelist said "We're never gonna learn about how safe the vaccine is until we start giving it." Said panel member Dr. Eric Rubin: "That's just the way it goes."[33] No Dr. Rubin ... that is not the way it goes.[34] When you ignore safety, you tend to ignore whether the injection even works, and while the "science" is moving forward, unfortunately deluded technocrats are not.[35] The FDA stopped being a regulatory agency and became part of the other alphabet agencies to promote the "vaccine." They saw their role was to get a needle in every arm, in everyone in every country—it was choreography to dance to the edicts of the DOD.

Pfizer now had the power to silence governments and maximize profits and power. Military bases, National Parks—just a few of the items signed over.[36] Big Tech and Pharma had bled out multiple governments to create this giant one world government monster with Pfizer calling the shots—literally. The human infestation would be eliminated with the silent, obedient consent of governments around the world.

## ORIGINAL ANTIGENIC SIN

But there were problems. The injection was killing too many too fast even though many of the injections were expired and ineffective (they were thawed for too long) and many blanks were shipped to many locations to mitigate the number of adverse events anticipated. Nevertheless, the body count increased, as well-hidden as those bodies may have been. They had to buffer the rollout of the injection because, again, it was supposed to have come on the scene after billions were already dead from CoV2 and few would be left to ask important questions.

One question was why give a non-sterilizing vaccine to everyone possible in the middle of a pandemic? ... All that would do is prolong the length of illness by pumping out a multitude of variants, which is exactly what took place. They were called variants because they had a different spike protein than the one the injection was having the human body manufacture, and so the efficacy of the injections started falling into the single digits.[37] This was all predicted well in advance, but the injections were pushed for socio-political reasons, not medical/scientific reasons. Compare and contrast what took place in Gibraltar v. Africa.

Africa is a heavy user of hydroxychloroquine (HCQ)—it's taken by millions. By the end of 2021, the vaccination rates in twenty African countries weren't even close to coming out of the single digits. Overall the African vaccination rate was around 6 percent, but for some reason the "experts" were mystified as to why there was so little COVID in Africa.[38] On the other hand, perhaps the most vaccinated country on the planet was Gibraltar, where there is a 100 percent vaccination rate, and yet cases of COVID were so high that Christmas 2021 was canceled. Unintentionally, they proved boosters don't work. In Singapore, with a 94 percent vaccination rate, cases and mortality spiked to record levels, and in Ireland, where 92 percent of the adult population is vaccinated, cases and mortality doubled.[39] The United Kingdom seemed to keep accurate records of its deaths by vaccination status (at least they did for a while). The COVID vaccines used in England (mRNA and DNA vector vaccines from Pfizer, Moderna, and Astrazenica) did not significantly reduce COVID mortality, but *did result* in greatly *increased* all-cause mortality.[40] Specifically in the United Kingdom, if you are under sixty and you get injected, you are twice as likely to die. As the months went by, the mortality of the injected only increased.

The mortality from COVID in an African country, such as Zaire, was 0.6 per 100,000. Almost no one received the injection. In the United States, the mortality was 1000 per 100,000. There should be no need to read one more word if you understand the obvious implications of that last sentence. Even before President Trump announced he had taken HCQ, the drug was disappearing and countries were removing it from over-the-counter status and requiring prescriptions. Someone didn't want HCQ to be around, and studies were being conducted with near lethal doses of HCQ in late-stage patients (no zinc, no azithromycin)—it was as if someone deliberately wanted to destroy any chance HCQ might have to help treat COVID patients. Then, perhaps one of the most momentous medical frauds in history took place —both the *New England Journal of Medicine* and *The Lancet* simultaneously published completely fabricated, fictional articles that concluded HCQ was not efficacious. What someone(s) had the power to fund fraudulent studies, compromise the world's top medical journals, and then get the FDA to pull the emergency use authorization (EUA) for HCQ? Apparently, that was the FTX group. Even after the papers were retracted, the FDA did not reinstate the EUA. This reinforces the problem that there is no FDA—the DOD took over the FDA regarding all things COVID.

However, those who successfully destroyed the possibility of using HCQ for COVID weren't done—they went after ivermectin, but not with the same success. First and foremost, data from nineteen countries that participated in the World Health Organization (WHO)-sponsored African Programmed for Onchocerciasis Control (APOC), from 1995 until 2015, were compared with thirty-five non-APOC countries —in other words, APOC countries are on ivermectin. That may be why they had almost a 30 percent lower mortality from COVID than non-APOC countries.[41] But what took place in India was even better. Two provinces took opposite stands. Tamal Nadu followed WHO recommendations and had the same dismal stats that the United States had, but Uttar Pradesh supplied ivermectin to its population and 97 percent of the cases were eliminated. Uttar Pradesh has two-thirds the population of the United States.

Despite the data on ivermectin, leaders from Australia to Austria actually believed the COVID injections worked and the unvaccinated were spreading CoV2—they probably still believe it, because they do not like to admit they were wrong. Ignore the fact there are no unvaccinated people in Gibraltar. Are these leaders psychotic or following orders from the Fauci/Francis Collins/Bill Gates/Bio-Pharmaceutical-Military complex? They wanted us to panic with each new variant, so they could continue to lock-down, have their digital ID's, take people to camps, and have the ability to inject humanity multiple times a year forever[42] ... that was always the plan. This was not the greatest public health disaster the United States had ever seen; this was done on purpose. But when events deviated from what was projected, the cabal scrambled to salvage the situation as best they could. So, insane medical rituals that had no foundation in science or medicine were pushed—the less than worthless cloth masks, the quarantining of healthy asymptomatic adults and children, and the meaningless six-feet social distancing guidelines (they pulled that out of their rear-ends). Remember, those that expired were very old, fat, and had multiple medical problems. There was never any credible reason to keep children from attending school and most lost two full years of education they will never be able to make up. Suicides increased, along with obesity and delays in treatment for medical problems that cost lives. The burden was on the poor who didn't have jobs where they could work from home, while the elite rich got richer.

It doesn't take a degree in immunology to understand that if you occupy the body's immune system making a spike protein that is no longer connected to the circulating variant, not only is the vaccine worthless, but it also perniciously lowers one's ability to deal with the actual viral infection one may get in the real world, because one's immune system is busy making antibodies to something that is not present and may be oblivious to an actual virus invading the body. The CoV2 infection has a very low risk of myocarditis, but it is there. The injection had the body make massive amounts of spike protein, and the amounts the injection was having the body make caused significant myopericarditis. The FDA actually asked that prospective studies be done, but they were never done by manufacturers. One such study has the actual risk at about 2.8 percent, or about three people out of every hundred. Conservative estimates have the risk at 1:<2000 (for context the Swine flu vaccine from the late seventies was pulled when it was found the risk of neurological disorder Guillain-Barre was 1:100,000.)

The population continued to be told "Safe and Effective" and the usual "one in a million (side-effects)." There was twenty years of data showing coronaviruses can cause heart disease, so one case of myocarditis should have shut the "vaccine" program down. But instead of pulling the vaccine, the CDC went to work pushing the idea that the "vaccine"-induced myocarditis was mild. It is just that there is no such thing as mild myocarditis; in fact 20 percent of those that die within a day of receiving the "vaccine" have myocarditis.[43] There is only one solution … immediately end the worldwide vaccination program and try to help people repair their immune systems. But compromised, well-paid "experts" will never acknowledge this solution. There is just too much money to be made giving everyone more "vaccines."

There is this insane group-think that needs to be overcome, because there are people in government, medicine, and academia that have been so indoctrinated to believe that if something is a vaccine, it is safe and effective—end of story—and they shut out objective reality at all costs. Even the government's own vaccine adverse event reporting system (VAERS) produced a massive death safety signal. VAERS, which is recognized for underreporting adverse events by ninety-nine-fold, still produced a massive death safety signal, but between the corruption and group think it was ignored.

The response to this inconvenient data was to order people to get more and more worthless injections that would do nothing but cause side-effects. Yet the presence of so many un-injected showed how robust natural immunity is; still, promoting natural immunity could put one on a terrorist watch list. They needed as many as possible to be injected as often as possible before the public became aware of the hidden sequalae of the injections. The control group had to be eliminated, or rounded up and terminated—at least that is what they wanted to happen.

Obviously, this story is not over. On their way out, the globalists will do whatever they think they can get away with to undermine and collapse civilization, including more bioweapons; they know their future is bleak and would sooner take as many with them as possible. But all stories end sooner or later, and when the story of the New World Order ends, it will look nothing like what its proponents had in mind. So, fight for freedom of knowledge, and in place of deceit, intolerance, and prejudice, fight for the possibilities of understanding, truth, and acceptance. For that is the reality humanity is moving toward, no matter how hard those who dish out their cruelties try and stop this change. Change is inevitable—it is the only universal constant.

# Introduction to the First Edition *(Incurable Me)*, Newly Revised

The greatest advancement in public health in the last 150 years has been sanitation, namely, clean drinking water and flushed sewer systems. Antibiotics probably rank second. However, the Centers for Disease Control (CDC) will tell you vaccines and fluoridated water were the greatest advancements—more to be said about the CDC later.

It certainly makes one pause to find out the lead contamination of the Flint, Michigan, water supply, at levels multiple times of what would be considered hazardous waste, was known for two years before anyone did anything about it. The Environmental Protection Agency (EPA) of the United States knew about it for almost a year before something was done. Was this willful criminal negligence? Let's say this event was just due to human stupidity, though the conspiracy cynic in me has some doubt. Maybe they were all drinking the lead-contaminated (and who knows what other contaminants) Flint river water, so they had a good reason to be so stupid. Who are they? How about Department of Health and Human Services officials, Department of Environmental Quality officials, and a bus load of epidemiologists. All denied there was a problem and insisted the water was safe.

It is hard to believe so many people can be so stupid, and let's face it, they weren't all drinking the brown Flint water, but they sure were drinking the "Kool-Aid." Was Flint a depopulation experiment? Did the depopulation lobby want to find out how long would it take people and governmental bureaucracy to react to being poisoned? There is no evidence for that; nevertheless, even if this was not intentional they still got their answer . . . two years.

Before you say you would never have let this happen in your community, taste your fluoridated water. Most of the fluoride added to municipal drinking water in the United States is purchased from China, and is contaminated with heavy metals. In a letter published in the *Cumberland Times-News* in 2010, Bernard Miltenberger, president of the Pure Water Committee of Western Maryland, said the bags of fluoride were found to contain lead levels of 40 milligrams per bag and arsenic levels of 50 milligrams per bag. Fluoride is actually more poisonous than lead, and when you mix all three heavy metals together the synergy between them logarithmically increases their toxicity.

But what does it mean to add 50 milligrams of arsenic to the water supply per bag of fluoride? The California EPA states four parts per trillion of arsenic will cause one case of bladder or lung cancer per million consumers, but that 50 milligrams per bag brings the level up to parts per billion—a 1000 times higher than the level known to cause cancer.

Now, if we are to assume that what happened in Flint was not some nefarious plot, then what is the culture the drives this type of devolution in health that is taking place today? Is it about not rocking the boat? Is it about doing everything to maintain the status quo and not call attention to yourself, especially if your career is in a regulatory agency with political appointees and industry insiders in high positions?

If you acknowledge the water pulled from the Flint river is corrosive, you are also acknowledging that not only was the decision to use that water supply ill conceived, but you are calling attention to the river itself that should be cleaned up, and that has more financial implications than just replacing lead soldered pipes. Then the lawsuits for destroying the health of so many . . . what a bureaucratic mess! As a career bureaucrat, that is not news you want traced to you. Alas, career security is often the number one priority, even though the truth is that there is no security in maintaining the status quo.

## PROFOUND DISAPPOINTMENT

The public has a profound disappointment with conventional medicine, which is the predominant form of medicine practiced today that does everything it can to maintain the status quo. The word *conventional* is being used here in its most pejorative aspect, that is, the over concern with what is generally held to be acceptable even if that which is held acceptable should be unacceptable. It is unacceptable to allow profit and share-holder value to dictate medical care. The Rockefeller Foundation birthed today's conventional medicine a century ago to facilitate the use of patented medicines in which those connected with the foundation had a financial stake. That is one reason why medicine is a business first and foremost. One need not look further than all the money spent on alternative therapists and therapies to get a sense of that disappointment—chiropractors, acupuncturists, naturopaths, hydro-therapists and homeopaths, to name a few, gives one some idea how much mainstream medicine has lost control of the population, but that is also a time when desperate measures could be taken to regain that control.

Things have gone so wrong in conventional health care and the practice of conventional medicine that if readers only take from this book an understanding that we have been put into a position of having to become our own healers, then something useful will have been accomplished. No longer can we assume that hospitals and physicians, regardless of how well intentioned, know what they need to in order to help us navigate our medical issues.

There are so many discoveries that have been made that could help so many. For example, the drug baclofen ($\beta$-[4-chlorophenyl]-$\gamma$-aminobutyric acid) has been shown to cause an effortless decrease or suppression of alcohol craving when it is prescribed with no limit of dose—meaning the dose needs to be increased as per the needs of the individual or it may not work. But work it does if a sliding dose protocol is followed. Naysayers, those that either won't profit by the acceptance of a new mode of treatment or will lose money if it were adopted, will submit we don't have enough randomized controlled trials (RCTs) to recommend baclofen to treat alcoholism. The problem is when a drug costs only a couple of pennies and is off-patent, then it is hard to fund multiple RCTs because these studies are very expensive. So the discovery that baclofen helps alcoholism and other addictions, for that matter, is not public knowledge and does not get translated into clinical practice.[44]

Is baclofen the answer for every alcoholic? Perhaps not, but then is there any medical treatment that works 100 percent of the time in 100 percent of the people it is given to? Alcoholics who successfully remain sober for years and decades often have to deal with cravings, but imagine if they did not have to deal with those cravings. How much easier their lives might be. The need to help addicts mitigate the untoward damage their illness is causing is pressing, and yet helping them with the chemical issues in their brains that could provide major relief is not an option even considered.

Cannabidiol or CBD is one of more than 400 active ingredients in the drug cannabis, also known as marijuana. It is also present in hemp. It is 100 percent legal, is considered non-psychoactive, and has been shown to help the brain deal with addictions in both animals and humans. The combination of baclofen and CBDs together are a powerful intervention not yet utilized, because this is not knowledge embraced by those who set the "standard of care" in addiction medicine. Addiction is just one issue where perhaps the most powerful medical interventions that could help patients are just not considered in clinical practice.

A decade after the publication of this book, perhaps it will be generally accepted that Alzheimer's disease is an infection with spirochetes, that Crohn's disease is an infection with mycobacterium, myasthenia gravis is a viral infection, and rheumatoid arthritis and sarcoidosis are often infections with mycoplasma.

However, today (2016) both ego and apathy, along with a lack of accountability, are keeping critical discoveries From getting translated into the clinical practice of medicine. Do you think the same groups that want to cull the population by 90 percent care about anything that might improve your life? The evidence is already in the medical literature for how to treat many of our most troubling diseases yet the same old attitude keeps on keeping on and we all suffer from the result. Is it possible that the paradigm of conventional medicine is holding the minds of conventional physicians in a place where they have lost the discernment to even know what they don't know?

It is human nature not to want to be taken out of our comfort zone even if that zone is very comfortable. Be it fear of the unknown or some false sense of psychological security, knowing that that one has always know and seeing only what one is accustomed to seeing is very comforting. But the cost of this faux security is the loss of an ability to admit that there are matters that one has no knowledge of – a closed mind is like a steel trap. Some, who do not have our best interests at heart, know that conventional medicine is a trap for some our best and brightest and are eager to take advantage of this level of control.

## THE HEALER WITHIN

It is a lot to ask someone who is not trained in the medical field to take on the responsibility of moving out of their comfort zone, but don't look to the FDA/CDC/NIH for what you need—they made that clear enough during COVID. Don't look for help from big pharmaceutical corporations; they are just trying to sell you something. For example, Pfizer never tested their jab to see if it would stop transmission—they didn't care. Don't look for help from third party payers; they are not there to help us as much as we might want to think they are—they just follow governmental and military edicts. And the internet is trolled and monitored by those with agendas to keep us in our place so shareholder value can be maximizes regardless of the damage done to others.

Much has been written about the waste in medicine from diagnostic errors, unnecessary services to fraud.[45] Not exactly an institution that instills the kind of confidence one would like given the life and death decision in its hands. In many ways it would be better if we could have taken back the responsibility for our medical care. If nothing else, to at least wake up to the peril of pervasive illnesses that aren't being acknowledged or treated. (*Did we really need some top-down techno-security state order to only use the drug Remdesivir and a ventilator to treat COVID patients? Of course, there was compliance because the government paid hospitals to only use those two modalities. But why? Unless they knew this tactic would kill and they wanted deaths along with the profits.*)

## Borreliosis

Lyme disease, or Borreliosis, has been with humanity for a very long time. The first known case was that of Ötzi the Iceman—a frozen mummy discovered in 1991 in the Eastern Alps. He only had to wait 5,300 years for the correct diagnosis. He was in his mid-forties at the time of his death, stood about 5 feet 2 inches, had hardening of the arteries and arthritis and, given his Lyme disease may have been the cause of all his ailments, maybe it was his physician who shot him in the back with an arrow—to put him out of his misery.

Fast-forward five millennia, we find this very nasty infection, perhaps as old as the Alps, has now found its way into the bone marrow of millions upon millions of Earth's human residents and few will ever know about it. Millions have no idea that their chronic debilitation, but usually non-fatal diagnoses—from ADD to chronic fatigue syndrome—may be warnings of this infection.

Other Lyme victims have serious cognitive issues, autoimmune disorders, and psychiatric symptoms such as anxiety, bipolar depression, and schizophrenia. Others are outright killed by the infection, such as with Lyme myocarditis.

If the current state of idiocrasy in medicine continues, the vast majority of these human victims will be neither tested nor treated for Lyme. How many victims are we talking about? I cite that figure in the chapter *House of Lyme*. It may astound you and push the most liberal calculations almost beyond credulity. A hint: in 2011, a scientific paper was published—a meta-analysis—that looked at the many studies published on the autopsied brains of Alzheimer's disease victims. Over 90 percent of these brains were infected with a spirochete-type bacterium, and in over 25 percent of the brains those spirochetes were for a single species of the Lyme spirochete.

*Borrelia burgdorferi* (Bb) *sensu lato* (sl) complex is the umbrella for a couple of dozen other genospecies. In Europe, several of these are pathogenic to humans while the pathogenicity of others is not yet fully understood. Genospecies of the Borrelia vary by location; for example, in the San Francisco Bay area, almost half the infected ticks will have B. miyamotoi (a genospecies in the Borrelia Relapsing Fever Group); whereas, B. lusitaniae is seen more around the Mediterranean basin.

The revelation that so much of Alzheimer's disease could be due to a Borrelia infection should have sounded alarms at the Centers for Disease Control and Prevention (CDC), but it did not. The CDC is not the organization most think it is. In March 2014, the director of the US Office of Research Integrity (ORI), David Wright, quit his job and issued a searing letter claiming pervasive scientific misconduct in biomedical research at the CDC, the National Institutes of Health (NIH), and the Public Health Service (PHS)—all part of Health and Human Services (HHS), which he characterizes as "a remarkably dysfunctional bureaucracy."

## CDC OFF CENTER

The CDC's image as an independent watchdog over public health has given it enormous prestige and its recommendations are occasionally enforced by law. Despite the agency's claim that they do not receive commercial support, the CDC receives millions in industry gifts and funding both directly and indirectly, which should raise questions about the science it cites, the clinical guidelines it promotes, and the money it is taking. But isn't the media an important watchdog—the fourth estate?

In a non-election year, 70 percent of the news media advertising revenues are from pharmaceutical companies, and if those companies don't want a story to get airtime, then that story won't exist. On the other hand, if pharmaceutical companies want the news media to run a certain story, they probably will.

The average person is not aware of the levels of incompetence and corruption that exist and persist in our most trusted agencies, and the controlled media is the last place to turn for information about what is really taking place. When it comes to Lyme disease, for example, an alarm should have been raised when, in 2014, the CDC said the true number of new cases of Lyme each year in the United States was 300,000, not 3000, but in 2015 the only ones ringing the alarm bell were the 6,000 members of the Entomological Society of America who found that "environmental, ecological, sociological and human demographic factors [have] created a near '*perfect storm*' leading to more ticks in more places throughout North America." (italics added).(5)

## LYME AND LYME AGAIN, BUT IT IS SO MUCH MORE THAN JUST LYME

The loss of human productivity, the mental illness, the suffering—all from this underappreciated, under-recognized, pernicious infection that somehow became an economic-political football between various academics, researchers, and funding sources. Lyme just became another gravy train for obtaining large grants that never advance our knowledge, because the intention is to just get another grant, not actually solve a problem.

If I am to believe the stories my patients tell me, there are still physicians at our most prestigious institutions who don't even believe there is such a thing as Lyme in any form.

If most people were asked, "If you had to have one of two diseases, Lyme or syphilis, which would you choose?" most would choose Lyme rather than the notoriously venereal syphilis. Both are spirochete bacterial illnesses. But syphilis is easily dispatched with antibiotics; Lyme, however, is not. If having

syphilis seems abhorrent, then having Lyme—which can be sexually transmitted as well—should at least be equally abhorrent. In a sense, Lyme is syphilis on
steroids.

Today, infectious diseases either are treated as a means for pharmaceutical
companies to make money or are ignored. If that disease does not fit into a model
where money can be made by pushing this or that drug or injection, then it seems
that no attention is paid to it whatsoever. In fact, Pharma no longer cares about
whether what they sell works, kills, or injures … they will sell it to you if they
can, even knowing it will cause harm—they simply don't care as long as they are
making money.

Be that as it may, we have a right to know what is making us sick. This book
is not a medical or legal treatise, but it is hoped readers will recognize that they
can no longer trust the usual conventional tried and true sources and must educate
themselves as best as they can. Remember the FDA wanted to hide the Pfizer
COVID documents for 75 years. It saddens me to say you can no longer trust your
own doctor, or anything you read in the media or the spew from governmental
agencies … they are all bought and sold, and if they can make money killing you,
they will. Yes, I know that is harsh, but that doesn't change the reality of this sad
situation.

Let's aim to facilitate the change in recognizing and treating the true causes
of so many illnesses that today go untreated or mistreated. The goal being a place
where the human species can continue to work with the incredible experience
being fully alive can provide, without the unnecessary burden of preventable or
treatable illnesses and without sick eugenicists releasing whatever agent they can
to cull the population. It is time to expose the death cult running interference with
our well-being and happiness.

I had a man in his seventies see me after struggling with idiopathic pulmonary fibrosis (IPF) for two years. This is a disease of the lungs that supposedly
has no known cause. It makes the lung tissue become thick and scarred so that
eventually you can't breathe; in other words, it is terminal. The prevalence may be
as high as 250 cases per 100,000 in the seventy-year-old set.

This man had seen all the specialists by the time he came to see me. I told him
IPF doesn't just come out of nowhere; there is a cause even if that cause has not
been established. I pointed out that laboratory studies support a potential therapeutic role for minocycline and antibiotic in IPF, which suggested to me that the
cause might be an infection.

Whenever I hear about an antibiotic healing a condition for which there is no
known cause, I think there is an infection driving the whole process. I put this man
on inhaled glutathione, a peptide the body uses to protect against oxidative stress

and remove toxins. Examination of his blood found a bacterium called Bartonella—the organism infamous for causing Cat Scratch Fever.

Bartonella is susceptible to minocycline, so one could postulate, as I am doing here, that IPF may be due to an occult infection, but today it is treated with immunosuppressants until the lungs can no longer be used and the patient expires.

One treats the infection and the mysterious illness that has no known cause gets better. There is a big picture here that should not be lost sight of ... on a societal level we have agreed to be unconscious about many things that are going on around us, in us, and to us. Besides the graft and criminal activity of big pharmaceutical companies (6), we have been rather unconscious about the food we eat, who created it, how it was made, and what is in it. Furthermore, we have made a decision to place trust in the hands of those who don't deserve it, and we do not hold those we trust to any reasonable standard of accountability. At the very least, we should impose a system of checks and balances that actually works to see if those given great responsibility are actually responsible.

Last, as you read this book, you will note there are omissions, such as any direct discussion about cancer, HIV, or the use of statins. These topics deserve a much more expanded forum. A small book like this has its limits. A book dedicated to Lyme by itself could be written here, so my apologies in advance if I do the topic an injustice or omit something important, especially realizing that many reading this book have Lyme and don't even know it.

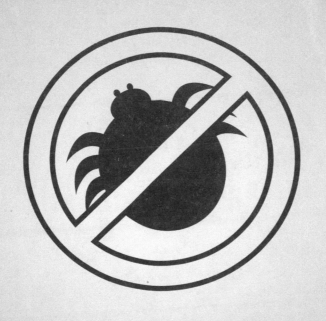

# 1

# The House of Lyme

*"Most men cannot accept even the simplest and most obvious truth if it be such as would oblige them to admit the falsity of conclusions which they have delighted in explaining to colleagues, which they have proudly taught to others, and which they have woven, thread by thread, into the fabric of their lives."*
—Leo Tolstoy (1828–1910)

Merely calling Lyme a plague doesn't do this pandemic justice.

Lyme disease ("Lyme") is unequivocally emblematic of how confused our society is and how compromised and incompetent our government agencies can be. It is right up there with building nuclear power plants on major subduction zone earthquake faults. Lyme is an unrecognized plague of vast proportions. It causes widespread damage to humanity. Lyme disease must come to the fore in the consciousness of all of us in order to end and prevent untold suffering for so many people.

It is possible to have empathy for the suffering of one or even a few individuals. It is not possible to take in the pathos of millions—that is just a statistic. And this plague involves millions.

It would certainly be nice if everyone could be given the secrets for curing Lyme disease and then treat themselves. The medical community in general isn't up to speed in its understanding about Lyme and can be almost as much of the problem as the bacteria. Then there is the societal disconnect from Nature, which is the problem beneath the problem. Regardless, for some ill people the potential complications of getting correctly treated can be so severe as to require both a medical coach and a caregiver. They must understand what to expect and how to receive help in what could be a rocky road to recovery. It is a nontrivial matter to get correctly diagnosed, and even more difficult to get correctly treated—even with all your support-system ducks in a row. This is a most difficult subject, but it is finally time for the light to shine on the house of Lyme.

## MY HOUSE OF LYME

In 1989 I was living in a quaint, 1,200-square-foot Craftsman-style house in sunny South Pasadena, California. The house was a few feet away from an elementary school where some very old trees were cut down. I could never figure out why there were so many ticks in those old trees, but they abandoned ship and dropped into my backyard. They were very happy to find the six dogs I was living with at the time. The dogs brought in only a few hundred of the thousands of ticks that had left the tree.

A few hundred adult ticks were fairly easy to find, as they were huge—but I didn't find them all. Several were mature females, who, having fed well from my dogs, were more than ready to create another generation of ticks. In addition to their abdomens swollen with recent feasts of blood (some of it mine), the engorged female ticks also carried ripe egg sacs. These mothers soon birthed what seemed like millions of super-tiny, flesh-colored baby ticks, called nymphs.

It was one of those up-close-and-personal experiences that turned me into a temporary tick removal expert. I suppose that is when I may have become infected, but it would be a couple of decades before I tested myself and learned I was positive for Lyme disease. I will never know for certain where, on the timeline of my life, I became infected. I am an example of someone who had minor medical issues but was never severely ill because my immune system is strong. I never had a "die-off" reaction to occasional antibiotics. I might have died never knowing I had been infected—even if it were the Lyme spirochete bacteria infection that eventually killed me, for example, by (faux) Alzheimer's disease. Others are not so fortunate.

Ticks are front and center in this chapter because the main organism in the United States that causes Lyme, *Borrelia burgdorferi*, is usually spread by ticks. Most who get bitten do not remember being bitten, and while it is hard not to notice being bitten by a large adult tick, the tiny nymphs often escape notice and literally get away with murder. They also bite more people than the large adult ticks if for no other reason then there are more of them.

The infamous bull's-eye rash that some get when a Lyme-carrying tick bites them doesn't show up on everyone. My theory is it shows up on those individuals who already have Lyme disease, making the three weeks or so of a single antibiotic that their physician may prescribe them an unfortunate undertreatment. There is more than one way to treat Lyme, but three weeks of a single antibiotic is not the way, even if one was recently bitten and didn't have Lyme before that recent bite.

## IS HYPERBARIC OXYGEN THERAPY
## THE PERFECT ANSWER FOR TREATING LYME?

I started treating Lyme disease patients soon after I opened a medical hyperbaric oxygen clinic in Santa Fe, New Mexico. In hyperbaric oxygen treatment, a patient receives oxygen under pressure as if he or she were a sailor in a submarine (see chapter 5). The Lyme spirochete bacterium is a facultative anaerobe, which means that although it tolerates oxygen, it really doesn't like it; in fact, enough oxygen will destroy the organism. How much is enough to destroy it? At least 160 mmHg (millimeters of mercury) pressure of oxygen—this is what we breathe into our lungs and a well-oxygenated bloodstream at sea level. But as oxygen filters deeper into our bodies, the actual oxygen saturation into the inner reaches drops significantly. By the time sea-level pressure oxygen gets into our bone marrow, the actual partial pressure has dropped to about 50 mmHg (mean pO2, or average partial pressure of oxygen)—about three quarters less oxygen than entered our lungs. There is even less oxygen reaching the synovial fluid inside our joints, and arthritis is a well-known Lyme symptom (although there can be many, many other symptoms of Lyme disease).

Hyperbaric oxygen therapy for treating Lyme can run into the same problem as antibiotics—biofilm. At high enough pressures, however, oxygen does penetrate biofilm, which will be discussed shortly. The presence of latent or dormant persister organisms of the Lyme bacteria, however, is as much an issue for hyperbaric oxygen therapy as it is for antibiotics. These cells are so metabolically inert that they can't easily be killed because they are literally dead to the world. They are the undead, and they can wake up if they sense there is no longer any threat. Hyperbaric oxygen alone is rarely the full answer, but it could be a big part of the answer if it were a treatment that was accessible to the public under the direction of a physician who knew how to use it in the treatment of Lyme. (Treatment is discussed at the end of the chapter.)

## "SHAMEFUL" LYME CONTROVERSY—DR. BURGDORFER

The whole subject of Lyme is steeped in controversy. For clarity, it is important to understand the back-story of this controversy. The disease is named after the town of Lyme, Connecticut, where the first documented cases in the United States were found in 1975. The organism causing the disease was isolated in 1981 by entomologist Dr. Willy Burgdorfer, who died at the end of 2014.

In the documentary film *Under Our Skin* (2008), Dr. Burgdorfer says, "The controversy in the Lyme disease research is a shameful affair, and I say this because the whole thing is politically tainted. Money goes to the same people who have for the last thirty years produced the same thing—nothing."

Lyme disease, if treated within a few days after a bite from an infected tick, is essentially curable with a single antibiotic (usually doxycycline for adults or amoxicillin for children) given for a few weeks. To be safe, it should be given for about eight weeks. However, there are more ways to get Lyme besides being bitten by an infected tick, and there is more than one *Borrelia* species that can be transmitted to humans. Lyme that is treated late or only partially, or that is chronic, can leave humans and animals extremely sick, often disabled, mentally ill, or dead.

## DIAGNOSIS CONFUSION? OR PROFITS?

The problem with the *Borrelia burgdorferi* (Bb) bacteria, as well as the controversy, starts immediately with diagnosis. Bb and its brother, sister, and cousin species all can cause Lyme disease. Some are very virulent, such as *Borrelia hermsii* (for the sake of simplicity I am calling any infection with a *Borrelia* "Lyme disease"). The bacteria are elusive. They try very hard to leave the well-oxygenated bloodstream for less-oxygenated tissues, such as bone marrow, the synovial fluid in joints, or the brain. Except in the relapsing fever varieties of *Borrelia* that seem to hide inside red blood cells as well, in general *Borrelia* prefers to leave the blood because it favors living in less oxygenated tissues. It is agreed that testing blood for the organism itself is not always accurate or completely reliable. (See PCR testing below.)

Blood testing for indirect immune system responses to the particular species of *Borrelia* is the only recognized means of diagnosis. But this is inherently problematic, because the testing is calibrated to match only the Bb group—not any of the additional related relapsing fever *Borrelia* species. In the San Francisco Bay Area of California, for example, *Borrelia miyamotoi* is probably as common as Bb. The current testing procedure also produces results that vary with the (usually unknown) stage of the disease, as well as the fluctuating immune status of the patient.

In 1994, the CDC and FDA gave their blessing to the diagnostic protocol that continues to be used today in 2016—a two-tier (two-step) diagnostic test based on measuring antibody response levels in blood. In the first step, called enzyme-linked immunoabsorbent assay (ELISA), antibodies responsive to a mixture of whole-cell Bb bacteria are evaluated—*burgdorferi* species only. Because some non-*Borrelia* microbes share some of these proteins, a more refined second-step test, the Western Blot, was implemented. This detects a narrower, supposedly more specific, set of antigen proteins.

| Spirochaetaceae | Treponema | | |
|---|---|---|---|
| | Borrelia | | |
| | | Relapsing Fever Group | B ___, B americana, B anserine, B coriaceae, B crocidurae, B duttonii, B hermsii, B lonestari, B miyamotoi, B parkeri, B persica, B rec-currentis, B sinica, B theileri, B turcica, B turicatae, B valaisiana, B texasensis |
| | | S. burgdorferi species-group | B afzelii, B americana, B andersonii, B bavariensis, B bissettii, B burgdorferi, B californiensis, B garinii, B japonica, B kurtenbachii, B lusitaniae, B sinica, B spielmanii, B tanukii, B turdi, B valaisiana |

Spirochaetaceae is the family of bacteria to which the spirochete Borrelia belongs. This phylogeny is still being explored and this diverse and pathologically dangerous group of organisms will undoubtedly grow as more discoveries come to the fore. They continue to corkscrew themselves into our bodies and under the radar of modern medicine despite the millions upon millions infected. The nameless Borrelia in the relapsing fever group is the organism Dr. Shah and I discovered in 2015. If it were up to me I would like to call it B shahnii.

The most contentious part of this two-tier diagnostic standard—some refer to it as the Dearborn criteria—is that it eliminates two key Bb proteins from the Western Blot test: outer surface proteins A and B (OspA and OspB). But antibodies to OspA and OspB are sometimes the only biomarkers present in those who have late-stage disease.

The CDC deals with this confusion by saying that their standard for testing positive, on the now truncated diagnostic criteria, is to meet the benchmark for case reporting, not for diagnosis. That is, if a lab finds a patient to be positive by the abbreviated testing, the lab has to report it just as they would if one tested positive for a venereal disease. But tell that to Lyme-illiterate physicians and insurance companies who don't want to reimburse if a patient doesn't meet the CDC standard (meant only for reporting purposes). Insurance companies continue to find it expedient to use the CDC standard as the basis for denying treatment coverage for all cases except the ones that labs must report.

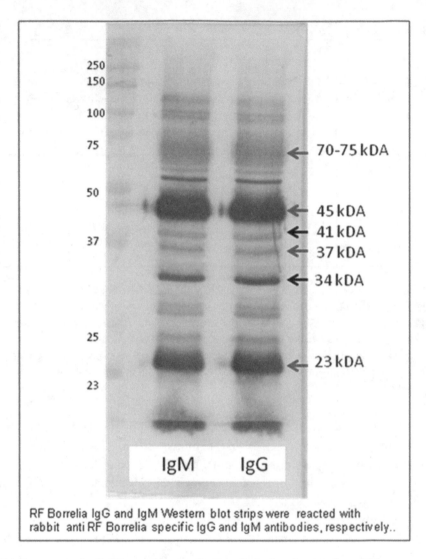

250
150
100
75
← 70-75 kDA
50
← 45 kDA
← 41 kDA
37
← 37 kDA
← 34 kDA
25
← 23 kDA
23

IgM    IgG

RF Borrelia IgG and IgM Western blot strips were reacted with rabbit anti RF Borrelia specific IgG and IgM antibodies, respectively..

This is an example of a Western blot test for *Borrelia* in the relapsing fever (RF) group. The organisms in the RF group will not test positive using the criteria for the *brugdorferii* group with or without band 31 and 34 (which is shown) included in the band count.

## THE TICK AND THE VACCINE

When LYMErix, the first approved Lyme vaccine, was given the green light by the FDA in 1998, Allen Steere, MD, was then chief of the Rheumatology and Immunology Department at Tufts School of Medicine in Boston. But even though Steere was in charge of the research that developed the vaccine, he seemed to have some reservations about LYMErix if given to individuals with the HLA-DR4 gene, which is present in roughly 30 percent of the population. Published in the journal *Science*[46] a few months after the vaccine was approved, Steere's evidence revealed a striking resemblance between a portion of the OspA molecule and the human protein LFA-1. LFA-1 is an *integrin*. It joins important white blood cells, called T cells, with cells that the immune system must act against: presenting the immune system with molecules or antigens the immune system needs to do something about. LFA-1, however, is more than just Velcro. It helps activate and program the immune system. Steere's concern was that T cells primed to attack OspA related to Lyme would also attack human cells lined with the "molecular mimic" and continue their attack on normal cells lined with LFA-1 merely because they look like cells lined with Lyme-caused OspA even if the Lyme-caused OspA were gone. The OspA antigen was the Lyme disease vaccine. OspB was the envisioned component of next-generation vaccines.

That is the mechanism involved in many untoward reactions that other vaccines have as well. Something in the vaccine too closely resembles necessary proteins or molecules in the human body, and the vaccine causes the immune system to attack parts of the body it should not be attacking—another reason why so many vaccines are inherently dangerous for many people, especially young children, even if vaccines were "clean" (free of mercury, aluminum, human DNA from fetal cells, retrovirus, etc.).

So, the LYMErix vaccine caused immune-toxicity in many of those who received it—a phenomenon where the vaccine sets the immune systems of the vaccine recipients on fire. Some people who received the vaccine became very ill with Lyme symptoms against which the vaccine was supposed to protect.

But in addition to immune-toxicity, there was another theory. The vaccine was given to many individuals who had previously had Lyme disease and were assumed to have been treated completely, usually by a standard (inadequate) course of antibiotics. But upon vaccination, not only did all their old symptoms reappear, but also antibody counts to most of the bands in the Western blot test unexpectedly soared high—bands that have nothing to do with the OspA antigen.

In all likelihood, injecting the OspA antigen signaled Lyme persister cells to wake up.[47] The previously infected Lyme patients, who thought they were free and clear of the illness, found themselves ill again with Lyme symptoms. *Borrelia* is not the only family of bacteria that create these metabolic dormant sleeper cells that wait for the right conditions to reactivate, but the presence of both biofilm and persister cells make treating Lyme a challenge for many.

Vaccine proponents and pharmaceutical companies were very upset that the vaccine trials were stopped in 2002, stating there was no justification for not continuing the trials.[48]

Nevertheless, in the real evidence-based world, it meant the vaccine may have reactivated a latent infection that either remained undiagnosed or was not completely eradicated in the individual in the first place and had returned with a vengeance. In truth, the situation was likely a combination of the above reasons—setting off an immune-toxicity reaction *and* activating a latent infection. If the latter is even half the truth, it means there are far more Lyme cases out there than previously realized.

## EVIDENCE-BASED MEDICINE VS. EMINENCE-BASED MEDICINE

The introduction to this book mentioned an article published in 2011, "Alzheimer's disease—a neurospirochetosis: Analysis of the evidence following Koch's and Hill's criteria,"[49] which is a meta-analysis, or literature review, of published studies on the autopsied brains of Alzheimer's disease (AD) patients. Spirochetes—the general spiral-shaped type of bacterium of both syphilis and *Borrelia*—were observed in the brain in more than 90 percent of AD cases. Bb was detected in the brain in 25.3 percent of the AD cases analyzed, and Bb was thirteen times more frequent in AD brains compared to control brains. The brains also had more than one species of spirochete—the infection was not just the cause of a single species of bacteria.

This bears repeating. Over 90 percent of AD brains had infections with multiple species of spirochetes, and over a quarter of these infections were Bb—the one particular species of *Borrelia* recognized as the main culprit in Lyme. That percentage does not drop to zero in the general population merely because most people are not diagnosed with AD. Kris Kristofferson, actor and country singer, has recently joined the ranks of those who are fortunate enough to find out that their misdiagnosed Alzheimer's disease is actually a *Borrelia* infection. What is the penetration of these spirochete infections in the general population? 20 percent? 40 percent? No one knows for sure, but it isn't zero. Why didn't this information set off alarms in all corridors of modern medicine?

The possibility that almost everyone with AD has a spirochetal bacteria brain infection is ignored, as much as most would ignore seeing a spaceship from another galaxy. It does not fit into the paradigm of our lives. We forget we saw the alien spaceship, or at least try to forget, and probably wouldn't want to talk about it either. Psychologists call this "cognitive dissonance"—when you know one thing but try to believe another.

Nevertheless, if these findings are correct (no one reputable has disputed them), it means that what we call Alzheimer's disease is *not* the incurable Alzheimer's most people think it is. Alzheimer's is the end result of chronic spirochete bacterial encephalitis—brain infection. Why doesn't the medical community acknowledge this revelation? It is an infection, so let us treat the infection.

A century ago, the bacteriologist Noguchi Hideyo, MD, demonstrated the presence of *Treponema pallidum* (syphilitic spirochete) in the brains of progressive paralysis patients (general paresis dementia), proving that the spirochete is the cause of the disease. General paresis dementia was eradicated after wonder drug penicillin was made available to civilian physicians at the end of World War II. Today, it is probably safe to say that no living physician in the United States has ever encountered spirochetal syphilitic dementia. Yet pathologist Alan B. MacDonald, MD, reports that he has found *Borrelia* spirochetes in the amyloid plaques of 100 out of 100 AD brains he has autopsied. It is history repeating itself in a sense, but MacDonald is just ignored—as did those who denied the existence of syphilis a hundred years ago. Amyloid plaques are abnormal tangles of proteins found in neurodegenerative disorders. Some believe this is the brain's way, albeit dysfunctional, of fighting off an infection.[50]

Whether it is denial or nihilism, many physicians believe Lyme is limited to a few select areas, and most areas are free of Lyme transmitting organisms. From Australia to Canada, many in healthcare ignore or avoid the reality of this infection altogether. For example, it has been over two decades since Wills and Barry (1991) found 42 percent of the ticks they evaluated in Australia had *Borrelia* in their guts: "These findings indicate that some species of tick often responsible for human and animal tick bites in this country commonly harbor *Borrelia* species spirochetes. On structural and antigenic grounds these microbes are likely to be the aetiological agents of Lyme disease in Australia."[51] Yet almost the entire medical community in Australia remains in complete denial.

## IF YOU HAVE THE MONEY, I HAVE THE LYME: PHARMACEUTICAL PROFITS LINKED WITH US PATENT REVENUES?

Three US government agencies—the CDC, the NIH, and the DoD (Department of Defense)—own partial rights to revenue from many of the US patents identified as especially significant for Lyme disease vaccines and diagnostic tests. We think of our government as some neutral arbitrator that would never make policy decisions, especially not decisions that impact on the health and welfare of its citizens, just because the government has a financial stake in said policy. Could what is true and best for science, medicine, and patients with Lyme not be best for the financial interests of the government and the pharmaceutical companies with whom they are in too close relationship? In 2013, the *Journal of Law, Medicine & Ethics*[52] published a paper discussing the fallout from the deep institutional corruption in pharmaceutical companies. We don't like to think this is so, but corruption is what powers our government at the moment. In a land where money is speech, buying politicians and government officials is a handsomely profitable endeavor.

It has only been a couple of years since the CDC revised its estimate from 30,000 new cases of Lyme per year in the United States to more than 300,000 new cases of Lyme per year. Until two years ago, with far fewer government-acknowledged cases of Lyme, there were surely less reason for the government to spend money on translational research that had relevance for treatment, that is, research that is directly relevant to treating patients. Did the push for vaccines, which are profit-makers with no liability, come from pharmaceutical companies alone? Why would pharmaceutical companies invest in translational clinical research for an infection that can be treated with off-patent (unprofitable) existing medicines?

## MORE CONTROVERSY

In the two-tier antibody-testing algorithm, the first-line screening test (ELISA) fails to detect up to 60 percent of infections. Patients who test positive are encouraged to do the second, more sensitive test (Western blot) if it has not already been done. The problem is that the criteria for *Borrelia* are so narrow in this testing that up to 90 percent of infected patients are excluded from being told they may be positive for Lyme or other species of *Borrelia*. That leaves countless numbers of Lyme patients who don't even know they have the disease because they were told they did not test positive, or didn't get tested at all.

What can be said? "Oh well"?

Significant differences of opinion on the prevalence of the infection are likely, which establishes itself in many who do not consider themselves sick or symptomatic (yet). At the risk that there will be those who will completely dismiss everything else written here from this point forward, a good guesstimate about the prevalence of *Borrelia* infections in the United States are numbers that range between 18 percent to 30 percent of the adult population. Some areas in India are seropositive, or infected, at a rate near 18 percent.[53] Lyme disease isn't on the radar in India anymore than in the United States despite such a large number of Indians infected. But what if 18 percent is a global infection rate for this organism?

In the Bay Area around San Francisco, I think it prudent to consider 30 percent of the adult population infected. North of the Bay Area, percentages are even higher, although those north of the Bay Area seem to fare a little better as the area is not as polluted, and people's immune systems are not so taxed. If we take the lower figure, 18 percent, we are looking at about 50 million people who have Lyme or one of its variations as an inactive (in remission) or active (symptomatic) infection. Can you imagine the uproar if 50 million Americans had syphilis and there were no consensus on how to treat it, let alone diagnose it? How could the CDC exonerate itself from culpability?

## LYME WORSE THAN SYPHILIS? SIMILAR TO TB?

Having Lyme disease is worse in our era than having syphilis. Why? Syphilis is an STD (sexually transmitted disease) able to be recognized early on by symptoms, diagnosed by blood testing, and treatable with antibiotics. With Lyme, however, not everyone gets seriously ill right away. There are those who can navigate through most of their lives with minor medical problems, never connecting them to show that Lyme might be behind them all. Unlike syphilis, Lyme does not cause you to develop ghastly ulcers on your private parts—a major red flag letting you know that you are infected. If Lyme were causing 50 million Americans to lose sphincter control or cause their skin to slough off, that would awaken the population. Lyme disease doesn't work that way. Yes, it is the cause of Alzheimer's disease, but again, that won't be accepted as fact for another decade.

Suppose you were a conscientious CDC employee in the Infectious Disease Division (which might require a lot of imagination). What would your options be for alerting the public about this pandemic other than to lie your little spirochete off and just keep things on the back burner? You just don't announce 100 million Americans may have an infection that is hard to diagnose, difficult to treat, and where there is no consensus on treatment and no test to determine if treatment was successful. That will just cause people to lose sleep, and when people lose sleep they grab pitchforks and come after you.

There are similarities between the Lyme epidemic and tuberculosis (TB) in our current era. Since TB and coughing were recognized as often connected, TB in the past was rarely an illness that could hide in plain sight. The TB epidemic of today is alive and well outside of the US and Canada, but over 90 percent of infected individuals are asymptomatic. Many with Lyme can remain fairly asymptomatic, too, if their immune systems are in good shape. But immune systems have good days and bad days, are weaker in young children, and tend to weaken with advancing age, so eventually most Lyme patients become symptomatic one way or another.

Diagnosing Lyme disease is nontrivial. It is possible to have not one single band positive on the conventional Western blot test and still have Lyme because the organism is capable of suppressing one's immune system so it doesn't respond. I was consulted on a little girl who had been diagnosed with rheumatoid arthritis since the age of two, but her Lyme results showed no antibody activity thanks to her rheumatologist who had her on immune suppressive drugs. The DNA of the organism was found in her blood. For many others, Lyme is a clinical diagnosis until the day when there is a reliable and acceptable direct test. That puts a lot of responsibility on clinicians who are currently mostly uneducated about Lyme and other *Borrelia* infections.

By relying on outdated CDC (dis)information, most physicians insist that Lyme is limited to a few select areas of the United States, and that most areas are free of *Borrelia*-transmitting ticks or other animal or insect vectors. They have no idea there are congenital or gestational transfer cases or that there is confirmed evidence that Lyme can be an STD. And don't hope that the blood banks' supplies are screened for *Borrelia*. They are not. If COVID taught us anything, it is you can't trust the Infectious Disease Division of the CDC.

The good news for the blood supply (relatively good news), and as mentioned before, this is not an organism (the *burgdorferi* group) that likes to remain in the blood. The yield from tests looking for DNA evidence that the organism is present in blood is as low as 30 percent positive even if Lyme exists in other body tissues. Some of Lyme's co-infections, however, like to live in the blood. Blood transfusion recipients could get infected with all sorts of things that aren't currently screened for, such as the protozoa *Babesia,* and a host of retrovirus contaminants. This is not some undisclosed risk from getting a blood transfusion or a conspiracy theory, as a *Wall Street Journal* article, "The Rising Risk of a Contaminated Blood Supply," revealed. The American Red Cross is currently participating in trials to see if new diagnostic techniques can screen out blood contaminated by *Babesia*, which is a protozoa parasite that can cause many types of symptoms. I would be remiss if I did not point out that the Borrelia in the Relapsing Fever group do like to hide inside red blood cells.

## INFECTIOUS DISEASE SOCIETY OF AMERICA GUIDELINES

The Infectious Disease Society of America (IDSA) periodically sets the guidelines for diagnosis and treatment of Lyme disease. These guidelines have not been updated to reflect the existence of chronic Lyme disease, of which evidence has been found in well over 300 peer-reviewed scientific journal articles.

The CDC benchmark on the Western blot test for *reporting* Lyme to the local health department has in effect been erroneously adopted as the benchmark for *diagnosing* Lyme, which is why positive test results are missed for up to 90 percent of patients. This is simply not a disease where you tell a patient you didn't make the cut as per the CDC so you don't have a *Borrelia* infection. It is a seriously bad mistake to make and I will always regret having made it myself in my early days of treating Lyme.

In 2013, the CDC announced that instead of 30,000 new Lyme cases annually, there were probably more like 300,000, and in 2015 they bumped it up to 330,000 new cases per year. This revised estimate of new cases per year was a pleasant turn toward reality by the CDC, but unfortunately their motivation for doing so may be less about accuracy and more about laying the groundwork for a pharmaceutical product that they have a vested interest in. While admitting their old estimate was one-tenth of what it should be, and the new estimate might seem like a lot, it may still be a gross underestimate if in fact one in six adult Americans has this disease.

To add salt to the wound of underreporting, the IDSA's guidelines recommend substandard care, which in turn creates a horde of chronic Lyme patients. The two-to-four weeks of the single antibiotic they receive based on those guidelines rarely cures them.

There is some good news. The more realistic guidelines of the International Lyme and Associated Disease Society (ILADS) have been adopted by the National Guidelines Clearinghouse (NGC) website based on the published work of Cameron, Johnson, and Maloney in 2014.[54] ILADS is a society of physicians and others who understand Lyme is not easy to diagnose, is not easy to treat, and can result in chronic, persistent infections.

The NGC is an initiative of the Agency for Healthcare Research and Quality (AHRQ), under the umbrella of the US Department of Health and Human Services. The NGC recently adopted the Institute of Medicine (IOM) standards for developing trustworthy guidelines, which define the highest level of excellence that a guideline can achieve. Guidelines posted on the NGC website must now satisfy these standards. Thus, the inclusion of ILADS's peer-reviewed guidelines on the NGC website demonstrates that the new guidelines meet the level of excellence called for by the IOM. Effectively (and fortunately for Lyme patients) it makes the IDSA guidelines no longer irrelevant.

In 2001, the white paper "Conflicts of Interest in Lyme Disease: Laboratory Testing, Vaccination and Treatment Guidelines by the Lyme Disease Association" documents how a handful of well-placed researchers with serious conflicts of interest corrupted the process of guideline development.[55] In 2013, Mary Beth Pfeiffer of the *Poughkeepsie Journal* found "ties that bind"[56] between government health officials and outside scientists in a disinformation campaign to steer the nation's perceptions and response to Lyme disease.

It is not that the individual physicians who signed onto the IDSA's guidelines don't believe there is chronic Lyme, as many have even published papers confirming its existence.[57]

When they all met together to set forth guidelines, however, conflicts of financial interests prevailed. In other words, these guys want to have their cake and eat it too. They want funding from the CDC and pharmaceutical companies, so officially they agree. But privately they reveal that not only do they acknowledge a different reality, they want to be recognized for what they officially deny. Can anyone prosecute them? This cognitive dissonance has cost many lives, and uncounted millions needlessly continue to suffer because some academicians want to maintain both their corrupt financial conflicts of interest and their scientific reputations.

Senator Richard Blumenthal,[58] as the attorney general of Connecticut, launched an investigation of the IDSA, based on allegations of abuses of monopoly power and exclusionary conduct in violation of antitrust law. In May 2008, Blumenthal said, "My office uncovered undisclosed financial interests held by several of the most powerful IDSA panelists. The IDSA's guideline panel improperly ignored or minimized consideration of alternative medical opinion and evidence regarding chronic Lyme disease, potentially raising serious questions about whether the recommendations reflected all relevant science."

In the article "Lyme Disease: The Next Decade,"[59] Stricker and Johnson said, "The review panel held a public hearing that featured more than 300 peer-reviewed articles and 1600 pages of analysis supporting the concept of persistent infection despite short-course antibiotic therapy of 2 to 4 weeks in patients with persistent Lyme disease symptoms. Despite this extensive evidence, the IDSA review panel voted unanimously to uphold the flawed Lyme guidelines."

The artificial Lyme disease controversy serves no one but pharmaceutical companies chasing vaccine profits and the corrupt, grant-dependent academicians they manipulate. There is an oligarchy of four pharmaceutical companies that control the $40 billion vaccine market, and that weight is more than enough to throw around to destroy any opposition; repress any impartial science; and deny, distort, and suppress the truth.

It took five years for the CDC to comply with journalist Kris Newby's Freedom of Information Act (FOIA) request for emails and résumés from three CDC employees. The emails, when they finally showed up, revealed that there was a shadow group setting Lyme disease policy, and a national research agenda without public oversight or transparency.[60] The group convened regularly online and during government-funded closed-door meetings. Aside from their significant ties to commercial interests in Lyme disease diagnostic tests and vaccines, this group made sure its members received the most government grants. The fact that it took five years to comply with the FOIA requests speaks to the level of collusion the CDC has with this shadow group.

## PLUM ISLAND—TEN MILES FROM LYME, CONNECTICUT

The last piece of the controversy concerns unexplained obfuscation around Lab 257,[61] which was part of a formerly secret Animal Disease Center on Plum Island a mere ten miles from Lyme, Connecticut. Whenever the government has had a hand in something nefarious, there always seems to be a lot of unexplained obfuscation.

In 1993 *Newsday* magazine found documents that proved the US Department of Agriculture had opened a secret Animal Disease Center facility on Plum Island in 1954 to create a livestock-based bioweapons program, although the government had denied it for decades. The Department of Homeland Security took control of the facility in 2003.

In 2008 an interesting article was published entitled "Wide Distribution of a High-Virulence *Borrelia burgdorferi* Clone in Europe and North America."[62] The authors of the study had determined that a Bb with an unnaturally strong virulence never seen before had arisen during the past two centuries. But when you understand that there seems to have been an attempt to weaponize Bb at the animal research facility on Plum Island (a bio-warfare research facility, despite what may be officially claimed), the timeline seems closer to the last fifty years.[63]

## HOW DOES ONE GET DIAGNOSED?

While it won't catch every case of Lyme, the best current testing is the Lyme Immunoblot panel, from IGeneX[64] Labs in Palo Alto, California. IGeneX add in the bands that were removed by the CDC (31 and 34) that connect to outer surface proteins A and B (their LTP1L panel covers both Lyme and the Relapsing Fever group). They report the results both as CDC and NYS (New York State) criteria and then again by their own standards that comprise these "extra" bands.

They can also do a Polymerase Chain Reaction (PCR) test looking for DNA of the organism. The yield from a blood sample on the PCR test is only about 30 percent even if you have Lyme. This is certainly confirmatory if positive (except to the CDC, ostensibly concerned with reporting purposes only). That potentially 70 percent high false-negative rate, however, makes getting the PCR testing problematic because of the expense. But there are many patients who will test positive only on the PCR. Maybe this is one of those areas where you are damned if you do and damned if you don't. Many of my patients are on immune suppressants because their rheumatologists are trying to turn off their immune systems, which is "standard of care" for rheumatoid arthritis, inflammatory bowel disease, myasthenia gravis, sarcoidosis, and others. They won't have any antibodies, so you either find the DNA or the organism itself on a slide or culture.

On the IGeneX Basic Lyme Panel, Western Blot, many patients will not produce enough antibodies to meet the benchmark of being positive (especially if the disease has been present for decades—the organism itself encourages the immune system to suppress a response to it). But IGeneX also reports the presence of sub-positive antibody levels—IND, or indeterminate, that is detectable antibodies but not at an amount to merit receiving a positive rating.

If the Western blot from IGeneX comes back IND or negative but there are antibodies for band 31—even only enough to earn an IND ranking—IGeneX can run an epitope qualitative immunoassay test on band 31. If a patient is positive on the band 31 epitope test, there is better than a 98 percent chance the person has chronic Lyme disease caused by Bb. The epitope test filters out cross-reacting antibodies from other sources that might cause a false positive (such as antibodies from the Epstein-Barr virus). Band 31 *is* the OspA of Bb—one of the two bands the CDC removed from diagnostic testing due to test interpretation concerns when the LYMErix vaccine came out.

It is possible to have a negative band 31 epitope (OspA) and still be shown to have Lyme by Western blot or PCR. A negative 31 epitope result means only that band 31 is positive because of non-Bb antibodies. To be clear about this, there is more than Bb out there: you can be infected with a non-Bb *Borrelia* species. You would still be sick, probably with another species of *Borrelia*, and should still be treated for *Borrelia*—for the relapsing fever group of *Borrelia* are no less troublesome that the *burgdorferi* group.

IGeneX and a lab called DNA Connexions will also do PCR testing on the urine, but as of this writing the rate of false negative results is unknown.

One last point here. People with robust immune systems may have much more positive and dramatic Western blot results than someone who has a compromised immune system from years of being infected, which is why there are seronegative patients who still have Lyme. Those with the most dramatic results are often the least sick to the point of not even knowing they are ill at all. Their immune systems have not been beaten back or beaten up by this infection so they are strong and mount a good antibody response.

## IGG AND IGM

The second to the last thing that needs to be said about the Western blot is that it can often reveal high antibody activity on IgM bands but not on IgG bands. Normally, when you get an infection, the IgM class of antibodies are the first responders, and the IgG class are chronic or convalescing antibodies. In Lyme disease either those roles are reversed or the frequent reactivation of the infection causes waves of IgM responses over time. The twist in this story, as already pointed out, is that there is more than *Borrelia* out there, and a Western blot or PCR looking for Bb is not going to find Bh (*hermsii*), Bm (*miyamotii*), etc. (IGeneX does have panels for the relapsing fever group.)

Immunoscience is the name of a lab that does a form of ELISA testing called Multi-Peptide ELISA (MPE) that seems to solve many of the inherent problems with the WB by utilizing in vivo (not in a test tube but in a living system) induced antigen technology (IVIAT) and enzyme linked immunosorbent assay (ELISA).[65] IVIAT is a technique that identifies pathogen antigens that are immunogenic and expressed in vivo during human infection. This test complements the Western blot, but neither is perfect.

If the above seems confusing, it is because it is confusing—far too confusing for most physicians to want to bother with, and there isn't anyone (especially the pharmaceutical company reps who most often directly convey information updates to physicians) helping them understand it.

But if you were to actually get diagnosed, then you have to deal with the really big challenge . . . getting treated correctly.

## EPSTEIN-BARR VIRUS, MYCOPLASMA, AND LYME

One of the challenges of getting treated is that Lyme interacts with other, separate infections, complicating diagnosis and treatment, so a brief word about Epstein-Barr virus (EBV). Almost everyone in the United States has been infected with EBV, the virus that causes mononucleosis and is responsible for a great deal of chronic fatigue. Many will never fully eradicate the virus and EBV often *reactivates* in the presence of Lyme and other infections. This is not an actual co-infection of Lyme, but a reactivation suggested by high antibody levels in a blood test, and should also be treated, usually by antiviral medicines. Some might argue that mycoplasma bacteria can be a co-infection, but the point is one is rarely just infected with Lyme—there are usually other infectious issues going on as well.

Since Alzheimer's disease is a neurospirochetosis, where did all these spirochetes come from to get into the brain? We know there are plenty of spirochetes that are present in the human mouth and within the gingival sulcus, or that area between tooth and gum tissue, so what if when infected with Lyme, the Bbs and associated genospecies start to interact with and modify oral spirochetes by exchanging plasmids (DNA strands that are outside the nucleus of the organism and can be exchanged between bacteria, like getting a postcard in the mail with instructions). Horizontal gene transfer with oral spirochetes could render these normally benign oral spirochetes much more virulent. Something to ponder for future research. . . .

## HOW TO GET TREATED APPROPRIATELY

Once you have a Lyme diagnosis, it is often a good idea to find a close friend or family member who can both guide and support you through the possible healing crises that await you. Not everyone has a difficult passage, but some have extremely difficult healing crises and need to be in a Lyme hospital; however, there is no such place yet.

Those who have neuro-Lyme (neuroborreliosis) are often so cognitively compromised or prone to any number of psychiatric symptoms that doing the right thing, being compliant, and "hanging in there" are nontrivial matters. Lyme can give patients schizoaffective disorder and full-blown schizophrenia, in which case almost all hope for progressing through treatment is lost unless there is a very strong friend or family member willing to work with such an individual.

## LYME PROTOCOLS

There are many roads to Rome (and somewhat fewer to Lyme, Connecticut). No one can claim they have either all the answers or a market on the best treatment modalities. I have been treating Lyme patients for well over a decade, and a protocol emerged that works for most of my patients most of the time. I do want to make the point that although antimicrobial warfare is not the only answer to treating Lyme (and so many ailments can be treated *without* blasting the patient with chemicals), if ever there were a reason to use antimicrobial agents, then Lyme would be such a time. Those who work with chronic Lyme patients would probably agree that biofilm, discussed earlier, is the rate-limiting step in treatment, that is, biofilm protects the organism and slows down efforts to get rid of the *Borrelia*. Persister cells that lay dormant biding their time are also a rate-limiting step.

I have patients who must start their treatment using only a small fraction of the dose of antibiotics I want them to be on. Their detoxification kinetics (their ability to handle toxins) has become so compromised that progress occurs slowly. There are those who unfortunately cannot go the antibiotic route, and there are alternatives, but they require more time, more diligence, and more planning.

Some of these alternative protocols include:

1) The Cowden Protocol;[66]
2) The Salt & Vitamin C Protocol;[67]
3) The Klinghardt Protocol;[68]
4) The Wolf-Dieter Storl Protocol;[69]
5) The Ross & Brooke Successful Treatment Recipe.[70]

I think there is something to learn from all the above, but I am not endorsing everything in any one of these alternatives. Again, I don't claim to have all the answers, and my recommended path isn't for 100 percent of Lyme patients 100 percent of the time. There are variations on a theme, far beyond the scope of a single chapter. There is hardly a month that goes by that I don't learn something new about this infection, so I am not presenting myself as an arrogant know-it-all by any means. I am sharing what works best for the vast majority of my patients, but that doesn't mean it is best for any one individual. This is a nontrivial subject with new insights and knowledge arriving all the time. Having said that, there is a lot of malarkey out there in a world where desperate patients have been abandoned and ignored.

You will find folks who swear up and down that whatever they are using is the golden ticket to get rid of Lyme. I don't want to be the pot calling the kettle black, but in examining one of the previously listed protocols—the Salt & Vitamin C Protocol—one can see why it may make certain patients feel better. Fourteen to 18 grams of salt and vitamin C will alkalize the body and make the internal metabolic environment of one's body inhospitable to many pathogenic organisms. But will it be enough to rid the body of the organism altogether? I think not. It is certainly enough to change the environment in the intestines to flush out many a parasite and worm, and while that is all very helpful, it is not going to eradicate Lyme bacteria in one's bone marrow.

I try to remain open and unbiased about nonpharmaceutical approaches, because anecdotal information for great interventions comes from them. I know there are very effective off-label treatments. After all, using hyperbaric oxygen to kill Lyme is clearly off-label, and yet it is one of the most effective non-pharmaceutical antibiotic interventions, perhaps exceeding all other interventions in both safety and efficacy for the eradication of the Lyme organism. But I have my bias about what will work and what won't. I own that bias.

## A BRIEF WORD ABOUT DIET

If you want to accelerate the healing process, stop consuming refined sugar, don't consume caffeine or alcohol, go on a gluten and dairy-free diet, and minimize complex carbohydrates. A paleo diet is probably a good model to use as long as you are not a vegetarian as a paleo diet is much more difficult to do as a vegetarian. Drink lots of water with a little lemon in it to keep your body alkalized. There is more about diet in the last chapter.

## BIOFILM AS THE ENEMY

Biofilm is the stuff you brush off your teeth. It is globs of adherent polysaccharide-based matrices that protect bacteria from the hostile host environment and facilitate persistent infection. Biofilms are responsible for a number of chronic infections from many types of organisms. They are not exclusive to Lyme any more than persister cells are exclusive to Lyme.

Antibiotics can't always get into biofilm. Even hyperbaric oxygen can't always penetrate biofilm, although it sure seems to get in deep. I have been able to evoke die-off reactions long after antibiotics are able to do so. It is biofilm that has been responsible for Lyme patients' requiring years of antibiotics, often only to suppress the infection, not eradicate it.

## HOW I TREAT LYME

Finding out that a relatively old drug, nitazoxanide, could rip apart biofilm, changed forever the way I treated Lyme. In the United States, it has a trade name as well, Alinia, and is approved to treat diarrhea from protozoal infections. Alinia is as close to a miracle drug as there ever was. I refer to it as an anti-invasion agent (not an antibiotic). It is capable of treating worms, protozoa, influenza, Hep B virus, and many intestinal bacteria (clostridia and *H. pylori*, to name two). It has also been found to have some effect treating ovarian cancer and colon cancer. This drug deserves a chapter unto itself, but the point is that this is the drug that has been missing from Lyme protocol: it has the extremely beneficial ability to address biofilm issues and it crosses the blood-brain barrier.

While it still requires the patient to have a functioning immune system, Alinia is so profoundly powerful (on the organisms that are sensitive to it) that I believe it is capable of dealing with Lyme all by itself in over 30 percent of the Lyme-infected population. Now, there will always be someone who has a bad reaction to the most benign herb, nutrient, or drug, so while it is possible to self-treat, there is always a risk. Although not the norm, not everyone can take Alinia. Furthermore, in the case of Lyme, successfully treating the infection also means the organisms will break apart and release toxins that set off inflammatory reactions, and in some people those reactions can be extreme. A novice will not know if he is having a reaction to the intervention, such as Alinia, or if he is having a reaction to the die-off of the organism.

This section is about informing what a possible best path would look like for most people. It is not about enabling someone without expertise in this arena to take matters completely into her or his own hands. That would not be wise, especially when using powerful interventions that have such a good chance of making a Lyme victim feel worse before it would make her or him feel better. I have some patients so chemically sensitive and so loaded with organisms that only a baby dose of Alinia can be used to initiate therapy. In some it can take months just to get up to the full dose.

If you are looking for a peer-reviewed article stating that Alinia can destroy the biofilm of *Borrelia*, you are not going to find it, but you will find articles stating that it destroys the biofilm of other bacteria, so what I did in my clinical practice is assume it would do the same with Lyme, and it seems it does—an understatement if there ever was one.

## THE HERX

The Jarisch-Herxheimer (Herx) Reaction (die-off) is a cytokine storm in which the immune system cannot distinguish between the need to set off an inflammatory reaction because there is a massive attack of growing infection or the death process of millions of pathologic organisms, which of course is a good thing. Because the immune system can't distinguish between the two, it is difficult for a patient to discern whether their reaction is negative or positive. If you don't have expertise, and you are the one in a million in whom a certain drug reacts poorly with your liver or kidneys, are you going to know? Or are you going to assume that this is a Herx reaction and you just have to bear with it? This is where supervision comes to the fore.

Proteolytic enzymes, such as serratiopeptidase (*Serratia* E-15 protease), are possible additions to the protocol in the hope that enough gets absorbed, and that what gets absorbed is enough to affect the Lyme biofilm. That is a lot to hope for; however, if Alinia can't be used, it is still worth hoping that proteolytic enzymes will attack the biofilm. The normal adult dose of Alinia is 500 mg twice a day, but there is nothing normal about treating this disease. If one is loaded to the gills with Lyme organisms, the Herx caused by 500 mg of Alinia twice a day could be intolerable. If an adult patient is having a severe die-off reaction, a dose of 75 mg or lower once a day may be more appropriate, and doses may need to be spaced out so that one takes the dose every other day for a time. Only tolerable Herx reactions warrant an increase in dose, up to 500 mg twice a day.

In some, Alinia causes sloppy-stool syndrome, and mass quantities of good bacteria (probiotics) are required to hold things together (it destroys the biofilm of *E. coli*). Causing bowels to move is not a bad side effect if there are a lot of toxins to clear, but in some, it can cause constipation, and mass quantities of omega-3 essential fatty acids—perhaps as much as ten grams every few hours—may be required. The omega-3 EFAs will do double-duty by mitigating the severity of any Herx reaction. Aloe, digestive enzymes, adequate hydration, magnesium citrate may all be needed to deal with severe constipation, but constipation must be resolved: it will cause a halt to treatment until bowels are moving. If constipation is still a problem, sometimes I will add the diabetic drug metformin (derived from the French lilac herb), which is an AMPK (AMP-activated protein kinase) activator that helps the cells of our body deal with stress, but it is infamous for causing loose stools. That might, however, be the solution for some people.

White sage tea (no more than one cup per day), saunas, and colonics are additional measures that may have to be taken to mitigate a severe Herx reaction. There are also absorbent resins, such as the prescription cholestyramine (don't get the "Light" version with aspartame [AminoSweet, previously known as

Nutrasweet] in it). Bentonite is clay consisting mostly of the mineral montmorillonite, and the medical-grade version is usually some combination of sodium and
calcium montmorillonite. In some patients the drug Trental (pentoxifylline) can
help with the inflammatory cytokines. Pentoxifylline and its metabolites improve
the flow properties of blood by decreasing its viscosity, so it is normally used
to treat peripheral arterial occlusion (a fancy name for a blocked artery in your
legs) that inhibits white blood cell adhesion and activation (because it affects the
inflammatory cytokines). It is not for someone with bleeding hemorrhoids, and,
like everything else, there are some who will be allergic to or intolerant of it.

Even before antimicrobial therapy is instituted, it might be an excellent idea to
get one's intestines in the best possible shape. A change in diet may be called for,
including elimination of gluten and other pro-inflammatory foods. The purpose of
the deluxe pretreatment preparation is to have a good idea if there are any foods
in one's diet to which one has an immunological sensitivity. There are several labs
that look at IgE, IgG, and IgA antibodies for several groupings of food antigens.
These tests have to be ordered from your naturopath, chiropractor, acupuncturist,
or integrative (MD) physician. That said, when one has serious infections, the
immune system can react or be sensitive to a lot of things it normally wouldn't
be, and getting rid of the infection takes care of those sensitivities as if they were
never there.

What about the infamous co-infections of *Babesia, Bartonella, Erlichea,* and
Rocky Mountain spotted fever? Well, the protocol described here should take care
of these party guests, so testing for them becomes somewhat academic. However,
if this protocol is not used, testing for them is mandatory. There is always the
possibility that one can have *Bartonella* or *Babesia* without getting Lyme. For
example, there are some parts of the country where almost all the cats have *Bartonella,* and that infection can be transmitted by fleas—no ticks required. So, just
remember that you don't have to have Lyme to have one of these other infections,
but someone needs to look for them to nail the diagnosis. There are also folks with
*Bartonella* infections that don't respond to the standard antibiotics and require a
little extra effort to eradicate, such as using the drug Mycobutin.

The next drug, an antibiotic, is doxycycline. Like Alinia, it has no trouble
crossing the blood-brain barrier and it has some antiprotozoal activity as well.
I used to prescribe it at triple the normal dose until I started using Alinia, but
since using Alinia, I dropped the adult dose back to the standard 100 mg twice a
day (best taken with food to avoid stomachaches, and those meals should be non-
dairy so as not to interfere with absorption). Alinia also is best taken with food to
increase its absorption.

The last antibiotic in the core part of this protocol is azithromycin, which has a nice synergy with doxycycline and Alinia. Here the dose is 250 mg once a day, and with all three on board and a good immune system, one could be looking at a mere two months of this protocol. But there's the rub—there is no outcome measure to use to objectively determine eradication. Now that we know there are persister cells that become dormant waiting for antibiotics to cease, then it might behoove all patients to pulse their antibiotics. If one is not having die-off and one completed a good first run—six to eight weeks—then the prudent thing to do based on the latest data, is to take an antibiotic holiday for a couple of weeks. Then restart the whole protocol all over for three to six weeks, and then take another drug holiday unless the first pulse produced no symptoms of a die-off. (This is the antibiotic equivalent to the "rinse and repeat" directions for shampoo.)

How long one stays on Alinia depends on whether there is a neuro-protozoal infection or a reactivated Epstein-Barr viral (EBV) infection. These infections take as long as a year, not weeks, to treat. Hepatitis B virus can be treated with Alinia, but a year of treatment is required. There is no reason to believe EBV would require any less time. The class of viruses that EBV belongs to can lie latent, waiting to sense that the immune system is having to deal with another infection, and then opportunistically take advantage of that surveillance distraction and reactivate. (More than Alinia is required to get rid of EBV—antiviral medicines are usually needed.) I would still pulse off of Alinia when the aim is to get rid of Lyme, but once it is decided that is accomplished, then comes the transition into an antiviral protocol, which is beyond the scope of this chapter.

There are some patients that are just better off staying on Alinia on a permanent basis because when they relapse the symptoms are serious, and suppression of the infection is the prudent thing to do even if that means staying on Alinia for years. Once one is convinced one no longer has an active infection then just taking quinine every day may be all that is required to keep persister cells persiter cells, that is, they don't become active.. Most people are alerted that they no longer have an active infection because their symptoms have resolved but Infecto Labs has a Borrelia specific cytokine test and if one has no elevated cytokines, one can correctly assume the infection is inactive.

Remember, when one gets Lyme, one rarely gets Lyme alone. Often one is dealing with multiple infections in multiple organs.

## ANTIFUNGALS

With all these antimicrobial agents, the chance of yeast (*Candida albicans*) overgrowth in the gut is high. For most that means getting a prescription antifungal medicine and taking it every other day or every third day. There is a very low toxicity alternative that some patients fighting chronic yeast infections have used, but it is not approved for human consumption—lufenuron, a chemical that is used in veterinary medicine. It interferes with the yeast's ability to form a cell wall. It actually fares better in terms of toxicity compared to human-approved antifungal agents, but again it is not approved for humans, and if you come across it (for your pet tiger [say no more]), make sure it is veterinary-medicine grade product. There are also herbal antifungal remedies, such as garlic (greatly underappreciated for its ability to fight bacteria, yeast, and virus).

I will most often use pulsed Diflucan (fluconazole) to keep potential yeast complications at a minimum. A small and unusual study was published in 2004 that is worth noting for the sake of completeness: "Clinical Effects of Fluconazole in Patients with Neuroborreliosis."[71] Patients were treated for twenty-five days after an unsuccessful run of antibiotics. Eight out of eleven patients seemed to recover from their borreliosis symptoms. A more plausible study[72] showed that the combination of doxycycline with fluconazole (Diflucan) decreased the biofilm of the yeast *Candida albicans* in the intestines.

While beyond the scope of this chapter, many patients deal with mold toxicity issues unrelated to being on antibiotics to treat their Lyme. Anyone with prolonged sinus problems, for example, may have fungal biofilm hanging out in one of their sinus cavities and, even more than antibiotics, what is needed are antifungal medicines.

Treatment for Lyme has to be individualized, and there are several variations on this theme. The bottom line when it comes to getting treated for Lyme is it can get complicated, and experienced medical supervision is required. Given that most MDs are still not up to speed on diagnosis (never mind treatment), this is a conundrum. I have provided information that will help readers understand what they are up against and what a possible path for treatment might look like, but for Lyme . . . You just can't do this yourself, as much as I might want to tell you such a feat were possible. It would be ill-advised.

Hyperbaric oxygen is addressed in chapter 5, and it has become a major component in how I treat Lyme in my own medical practice. It not only enhances the immune system but also acts directly as an antibiotic with organisms that cannot stand too much oxygen.

In 2013, the Woods Hole Oceanographic Institute in Massachusetts discovered that the *Borrelia* organism is manganese dependent because it substitutes manganese in place of where almost all other organisms use iron. By doing so, manganese helps the *Borrelia* evade the immune system. A second-tier antituberculosis drug called *para*-aminosalicylic acid (PAS, 4-aminosalicylic acid or 4-PAS) can bring down manganese levels in the human body and make life very tough for the Lyme bacteria, but there have been no clinical studies in this area, and PAS is not for everyone. Recently it was found that that the common OTC (over the counter; that is, nonprescription) antihistamine Claritin (loratadine) inhibits manganese transport into the Lyme organism. However, the study was a test-tube study (in vitro) and may not apply in a real-world situation at a dose where loratadine can be safely used. Many things work in vitro and have zero application in a living organism (in vivo). There is another drug that appears to be even more effective at dropping manganese levels: 5-ASA or 5-aminosalicylic acid (mesalamine).[73]

Ultimately, Lyme is still a clinical diagnosis that does not rely only on laboratory test findings. Some interesting biomarkers can guide in determining the length of treatment required, such as the CD 57 level, but these biomarkers are not perfect, and some patients never develop healthy CD 57 levels despite strong clinical evidence that they have weathered the infection and come out on top. Furthermore, one could have a healthy CD 57 level in the presence of a few dormant persister cells. This level of uncertainty about how and when to treat, how and when to stop treating, and the lack of lab testing that gives definitive answers is not conducive to having your average MD want to get involved. Only a functional medicine MD or DO who has a true interest in this area wants to treat Lyme patients.

## HERBS

Many Lyme patients, often because of the lack of support and knowledge in the conventional medical community, feel that herbs are the best way to treat this disease. I am very supportive of using and understanding botanical medicines, but I do not think they can work their magic consistently enough, in the case of Lyme. They should be considered supportive only.

Garlic[74] and oregano[75] are well known for their antimicrobial ability. This ability seems to inhibit quorum sensing, which is an ability to turn genes on or off depending on the density of other bacteria in the local environment. Phenolics such as thymol and carvacrol in oregano interact with surface proteins of bacteria, leading to an alteration of the cell surface and thereby compromising the initial attachment phase of biofilm formation. The rate-limiting step is whether any particular patient is willing to consistently take his or her herbal remedies in the quantity and frequency to eliminate the infection. Using these two herbs, garlic and oregano, which I would consider medicinal foods, can require the consumption of considerably large quantities of these herbs taken every few hours for months to accomplish one's aim—a task few could do successfully.

But, it can be done. I had to self-treat a persistent pseudomonas lung infection in the days before the antibiotic ciprofloxin. Treatment required bottles of garlic extract multiple times a day, but eventually I got rid of an infection that I had to deal with for months. Garlic is always my "go-to" herbal antimicrobial agent, with oregano oil a very close second.

There are other answers out there. The future will reveal perhaps even more aggressive protocols for antibiotic-resistant Lyme. In 2015, for example, a promising *in vitro* study was published that suggested that a combination of daptomycin in conjunction with doxycycline and cefoperazone might be effective for treating persistent Lyme.[76] But this is a test-tube study and needs to be further evaluated, as all test-tube studies do. In 2016, a study was published that indicated a certain antibiotic combination might work (*in vitro*) against perister cells[77] (artemisinin/cefoperazone/doxycycline and sulfachlorpyridazine/daptomycin/doxycycline). Because it is so well tolerated, I wish they had studied Alinia, but they did not.

As if Lyme weren't enough to deal with, on so many levels, there is more. Tacaribe virus is an arenavirus discovered in ticks. Until recently, it had never been found in an animal or human species in the United States. It is not known to cause disease in humans, but other members of this class cause several varieties of hemorrhagic fever. This virus is now in 10 percent of ticks collected in north central Florida.[78] In addition, the lethal Bourbon virus, which is an RNA[79] virus, has been found in one person so far in the United States; there is neither diagnostic testing nor official treatment for it. However, these rare viruses are good reasons to start all suspected tick-borne illness patients on Alinia, because Alinia is effective against influenza, which is also a member of this family of viruses. Again, there is no known effective treatment, but I would use a combination of Alinia and ribavirin, which stops RNA synthesis (it is also effective against DNA viruses).

The Powassan virus (a member of the *Flaviviridae* family) is also a tick-borne illness. There have been fewer than 100 documented cases in the United States in the last ten years, so it doesn't seem to be very common. But there is no question that Alinia has activity in the *Flaviviridae* class of viruses and should be used perhaps with ribavirin. It is worth noting that the Zika virus that is often accused of causing small heads, or microcephaly, with infants born to mothers who became infected during pregnancy also belongs to this class.

The above is mentioned in an attempt to be as quasi-comprehensive about Lyme and co-infections as possible in this single chapter, but it should be obvious now why I am such a strong advocate for using Alinia in this arena of infectious disease.

## DECREASE THE TICK POPULATION

To help decrease the tick population something should be done in a very proactive, environmentally friendly way, and that would be a liberal introduction of foxes into high tick-infested areas, as they will eat a lot of rodents that the ticks feed off. Where possible, introduce opossums, which will dine on the ticks themselves. Perhaps the most voracious tick eater I have learned about is the guineafowl or guineahen—a bird native to Africa. The helmeted guineafowl, as a wild bird, has been introduced in many locations. One of my patients told me that on her farm in Nebraska the bird reduced the tick population by 90 percent. But don't hold your breath waiting for this to be implemented until there is an honest accounting for how many of us are actually infected.

## THE HOMELESS

There is no reason to believe the homeless population is a reservoir of Bb, any-more than anyone else. They are certainly more vulnerable to a host of infections, such as, *Bartonella quintana* (trench fever). The dumping of patients from state mental hospitals a few decades ago created a caste system in our country where there was none before, and while one might ignore the unfortunates, it is not as easy to ignore an infectious disease that knows no caste. The safety net for vaga-bonds and the mentally ill that should have been created when mental hospitals were closed never materialized—another shame on us and American society.

## A BRIEF WORD ABOUT MORGELLONS DISEASE—COLLAGEN AND KERATIN VARIANT OF LYME DISEASE

In 2015 an article was published entitled "Exploring the association between Morgellons disease and Lyme disease: Identification of *Borrelia burgdorferi* in Morgellons disease patients."[80] This study looked at an unprecedented twenty-five patients who presented with Morgellons disease (MD), which is a complex dermopathy characterized by bizarre skin lesions that contain multicolored filaments either lying under, embedded in, or projecting from skin, along with a host of constitutional, musculoskeletal, and neurocognitive symptoms well known to Lyme victims. Despite overwhelming evidence to the contrary, MD continues to be attributed to delusions of parasitosis (delusional infestation with parasites) by the very few physicians who have even heard of it.

The authors of the study, Middelveen et al., detected *Borrelia* DNA by PCR and/or staining with Bb-specific DNA probes in twenty-four out of twenty-five patients and were able to culture viable Bb spirochetes from skin, blood and vaginal secretions of some patients. The presence of spirochetes was confirmed by numerous testing methodologies, including culture, histology, anti-Bb immunostaining, electron microscopy, PCR and in situ Bb-DNA hybridization.

The mysterious MD filaments are not textile fibers, as many believe. MD fibers are biofilaments produced by epithelial cells stemming from deeper layers of the epidermis and the root sheath of hair follicles. The "fibers" are the MD sufferers' own collagen and keratin.

Bb appears to attach to fibroblasts and keratinocytes; the intracellular sequestration of Bb in skin fibroblasts and keratinocytes may protect the spirochete from host defense mechanisms. There should be no doubt that MD is a true infectious illness variant of Lyme disease.

Despite many articles showing an association with *Borrelia* and MD, the "official" CDC position is that MD patients are in need of psychiatric help and that there is no evidence of an infection. The medical community owes the thousands of MD patients a giant apology. In lieu of that unlikely apology, I offer it in their stead. I have always treated MD patients as if they had Lyme. I was very glad to learn I did the right thing for those patients who came to me for help. Physicians don't know everything—I certainly don't—and I am not always right on the mark. While I try to get close, reality intervenes. Again, this group of patients should get some special type of dispensation from someone. They have been treated like excrement, and the physicians who have attempted to help them have often been run out of town.

I started using ivermectin topically mixed with tea tree oil and orally as well, as part of my protocol for treating MD.

The CDC's position on MD relies heavily on data from the Managed Care Organization in Northern California, Kaiser Permanente, where you won't even get the Western blot test for Lyme unless your ELISA is positive. In the real world, Lyme is a true pandemic. One day there will be an accounting for those whose ego- and greed-centered decisions have let the Lyme plague get so out of hand, literally causing death and destruction in its wake. More than a pandemic, this is the global medical negation of an illness. This is a Nuremberg Trial–level offense, but what follows in the next chapter makes Lyme look like child's play.

# 2

# Dementia: Are We All Getting Dicofo(o)l'ed?

*"If she herself had had any picture of the future, it had been of a society of animals set free from hunger and the whip, all equal, each working according to his capacity, the strong protecting the weak. . . . Instead—she did not know why—they had come to a time when no one dared speak his mind, when fierce, growling dogs roamed everywhere, and when you had to watch your comrades torn to pieces after confessing to shocking crimes."*

—George Orwell, *Animal Farm*, 1945

In the first chapter, the fickle finger of ego-driven hubris pointed toward a few nefarious types who may have been trying to weaponize Bb on Plum Island, New York. These include the usual suspects from the IDSA and the CDC regarding recognizing the severity of the disease, and its diagnostic and treatment dilemmas—medical crimes no matter how you slice them. The story about what is going on with dementia is even more disturbing and brings home a quandary we were all facing even before the COVID bioweapon.

According to the National Institute of Aging, "Alzheimer's disease is the most common cause of dementia among older people. Dementia is the loss of cognitive functioning—thinking, remembering, and reasoning—and behavioral abilities, to such an extent that it interferes with a person's daily life and activities."[81] The University of Michigan Health and Retirement Study (HRS) is a longitudinal panel study that every two years surveys a representative sample of more than 26,000 Americans over the age of fifty.[82] The results of this survey imply that well over half of adults over the age of seventy go undiagnosed and untreated. In the United States, more than five million people currently live with Alzheimer's disease (AD), including one in nine people greater than the age of sixty-five years.[83] Therefore, one could postulate that the true incidence is well over ten million Americans.

Based on the "2014 Report on the Milestones for the US National Plan to Address Alzheimer's Disease,"[84] there are three recognized stages of the disease: "(1) dementia due to Alzheimer's, (2) mild cognitive impairment (MCI) due to

Alzheimer's, and (3) preclinical (presymptomatic) Alzheimer's." A fourth stage would be Alzheimer's-related changes observed during an autopsy. According to Medicare data, 1 in 3 seniors who die in any given year were diagnosed with AD. An estimated 700,000 Americans over sixty-five died of AD[85] in 2015, based on the Chicago Health and Aging Project (CHAP). Ultimately, AD is not just a neuro-cognitive disorder but also a fatal, incurable disease. Or is it?

Officially, AD is a disease of unknown etiology. However, it is widely accepted that most AD is not directly genetically inherited and that some external vector, such as a toxicant exposure or an infection, must be involved for the disease to progress into a clinically observable condition.

If an infectious agent were involved, it seems as if it would have been identified by now. Indeed in 2011, the meta-analysis that was mentioned in the last chapter found bacteria called spirochetes in the brain in more than 90 percent of AD cases.[86] *Borrelia burgdorferi* was detected in the brain in 25.3 percent of AD cases analyzed and was thirteen times more frequent in AD compared to controls. Periodontal pathogenic *Treponema*[87] and *Borrelia burgdorferi* were detected using species-specific PCR and antibodies. Importantly, co-infection with several spirochetes occurs in AD.

## SO CLOSE AND YET SO FAR

In 2014, a randomized double-blind and controlled (RCT) trial[88] found that mino-cycline (brother of doxycycline) significantly improved the negative symptoms of schizophrenia. What received the credit were the known anti-inflammatory properties of minocycline, not that it might actually be treating an infection. This mistake gets repeated over and over in medicine—so close to the truth, but so far from reality. It is of interest to note that a 1994 map of the United States shows nearly identical geographic distributions of Lyme and schizophrenia.

If these research results were embraced, an obvious intervention would be to bring diagnostic testing to a much higher level of usefulness than exists today by screening widely for these organisms and then treating the infection(s) with protocols based on evidence, neither of which is done today. This would help those who have and will get Lyme disease and other opportunistic infections, as well as those at risk for dementia. There is reason why this is not happening and a reason under the reason.

In early 2014, in an article published in *JAMA Neurology*,[89] Rutgers scientists discuss their findings in which levels of DDE (dichlorodiphenyldichloroethylene) were higher in the blood of late-onset Alzheimer's disease patients compared to those without the disease. DDT (dichlorodiphenyltrichloroethane) doesn't break down to any great extent, but it will lose a hydrogen atom (hydrogen chloride, or

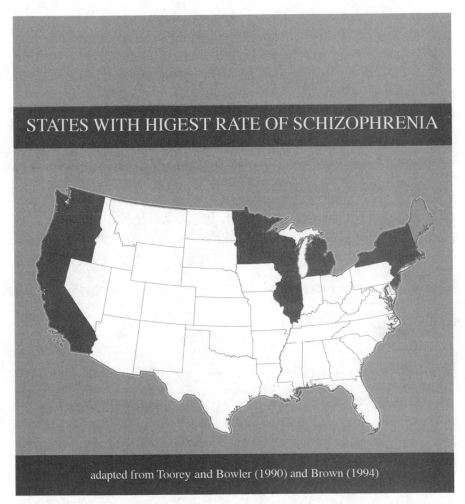

STATES WITH HIGEST RATE OF SCHIZOPHRENIA

adapted from Toorey and Bowler (1990) and Brown (1994)

From Brown JS Jr., "Geographic correlation of schizophrenia to ticks and tick-borne encephalitis." *Schizophrenia Bulletin* 1994; 20(4):755–75.

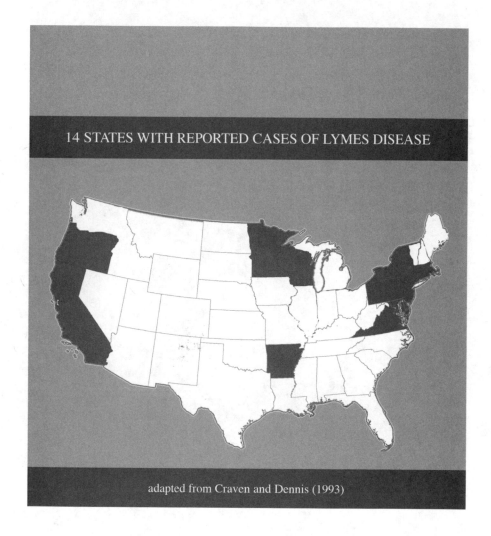

14 STATES WITH REPORTED CASES OF LYMES DISEASE

adapted from Craven and Dennis (1993)

HCL, to be exact). DDE is just as deadly and should just be considered another form of DDT.

A decade earlier the article "Neurodegenerative Diseases and Exposure to Pesticides in the Elderly" clearly showed that occupational pesticide exposure increased the incidence of AD and Parkinsonism. The point is that the connection between pesticide exposure and both human and animal diseases, especially neurological diseases, is not an unknown mystery or big surprise. Good thing DDT is banned!

But it is not banned—not even in the United States. Its use was cut back in the United States, but don't for one minute believe the manipulation and the illusion. The noxious effluvia that has been thrown at us just so that a few could profit. What we have is a catastrophic failure of the government to keep commercial sectors, in this case agribusiness, from polluting us, spying on us, and in this case controlling the food supply. It is immoral, it is odious, and it is essentially warfare on society for the profit of a few.

## A POISON BY ANY OTHER NAME

DDT is used in the United States to control insects in crops and livestock and to combat insect-borne diseases. It was introduced as a pesticide during WWII. In the United States, the general use moratorium took place in 1972, but now here comes the rub. Dicofol, which is made and sold by Dow AgroSciences and carries the trademark Kelthane, is DDT. In China dicofol is produced by the Yangzhou Pesticide Factory, which reports production quantities of four million pounds of dicofol per year. It is also produced in Brazil, India, and Spain.

Dicofol[90] is virtually identical to DDT, and in fact synthetic estrogens, such as ethinyl estradiol (EE2), have less in common with estrogen than dicofol has with DDT. Only one little hydroxyl group added to DDT turns it into dicofol. If DDT were a pig, dicofol would be that same pig with the smell of beer on its breath. The ban on DDT was all smoke and mirrors, and no one—no agency and even the Stockholm Convention—was willing to stand up for the citizens of this planet. No one in a position to do something stopped this, allowing the rest of us to be fooled—dicofo(o)led.

Rutgers scientists directly linked a specific chemical compound to Alzheimer's disease that is in DDT and DDE, and it is no great leap to postulate that DDT and DDE increase the incidence of neurospirochetosis by injuring the immune system that is already injured by other toxins and heavy metals. It is always more than one thing.

DDT

Dicofol

The chemical structure of the two virtually identical pesticides DDT and dicofol.

This bears repeating: DDT and DDE are directly linked to Alzheimer's disease. Not an association, not some vague possible causality—a direct link. Therefore, the conscious use of anything with DDT and DDE in it would be the deliberate use of a substance to cause harm.

There are other illnesses for which DDT/DDE are responsible.

This class of insecticide (organochlorides) impacts the electrical activity in the body, so it affects brain and heart, but there are other organs that also use electrical current, including the lungs. It clearly affects the immune system and causes cancer, and it doesn't break down in the environment.

In 2009, a study was published titled "Organochlorine and heavy metals in newborns: results from the Flemish Environment and Health Survey (2002–2006)"[91] in which "DDE and Pb were measurable in nearly all samples." That tells us that DDE has now become ubiquitous—it is everywhere and in everybody and is given to everyone so that shareholder value can be maximized. That is the only reason, for if this were just about insect control, there are alternatives. For example, in 2011, researchers published an article (Pedercini, et al., 2011)[92] showing that focus on non-DDT insecticide treated bed nets and environmental management show higher levels of cost effectiveness. Treated bed nets and environmental management would also allow phasing out DDT in a cost-effective manner in those parts of the world where it is still used with abandon to kill mosquitoes.[93] The Stockholm Convention on Persistent Organic Pollutants treaty, signed in 2001 and effective from May 2004, aims to eliminate or restrict the production and use of persistent organic pollutants (POPs). But DDT is not required to be eliminated—only restricted. DDT has friends in high places, and they insist it is still needed for disease vector control: malaria. Dicofol isn't even on the list even though it is essentially DDT (but for the addition of that little OH [hydroxyl] group.) Dicofol aside, DDT continues to be used with abandon. Ethiopia, South Africa, India, Mauritius, Myanmar, Yemen, Uganda, Mozambique, Swaziland, Zimbabwe, North Korea, Eritrea, Gambia, Namibia, and Zambia are all using DDT (not just dicofol, but straight DDT). Think about ten million pounds of DDT being sprayed in Africa per year alone. It makes those populations prone to both poliovirus-facilitated acquired flaccid paralysis (AFP),[94] as well as non-"polio" enterovirus, AFP. Think about those in control who want everyone to believe it is just all about a virus—a single virus.

The family of viruses that causes AFP belongs to the enterovirus (EV) family, but the immune system has to be compromised for them to wreak havoc in the nervous system. Just consider the possibility that the infamous "polio" epidemic was a man-made and provoked paralysis when a benign virus opportunistically took advantage of those with a compromised immune system because they were sub-clinically poisoned with pesticides. In 2006, the World Health Organization (WHO) changed its policy and told affected countries to use DDT—and they do. There are over 200 million cases of malaria worldwide and close to a million deaths. Well over 90 percent of all of this activity takes place in Africa, and children are disproportionally affected. This is a serious infection, but the fact is that no one is going to get rid of all the malaria vector mosquitoes (certainly not with DDT), and the use of DDT is not sustainable. So, where does that leave all of us?

There will always be those who think that DDT is indispensable to any malaria control program, because they will say it is so much less expensive and more effective, but that is propaganda. The truth is that treated bed nets and environmental management would also allow phasing out DDT in a cost-effective manner, because it is more effective in preventing malaria and less expensive than spraying DDT; therefore, DDT phase-out would only make logical medical and financial sense.

The bottom line is that using DDT is not a sustainable solution, and it is obviously having a significant impact on human health. Too many die of malaria today, but there is a lot of fallout from using DDT. It causes disease and misery that is not being factored into the equation (by those with good intentions or not). And then there is dicofol.

If it were acknowledged that DDT is responsible for Alzheimer's disease and is responsible for allowing the poliovirus as well as other entero-viral agents to be so destructive to the human central nervous system, you can bet DDT would not be allowed. It would be banned in the United States and listed for elimination by the Stockholm Convention. But the truth of DDT's dangers has been hidden from the public. If everyone knew the facts, none of this would be allowed. Here is but one example from an unclassified paper, "Studies of Biologically Active Agents in Cells and Tissue Cultures,"[95] from the US Army Medical Research and Development Command (with MIT): "Poliovirus infection. In the poliovirus experiments . . . it is evident that at the 20 and 40 μg levels of DDT, the yield of virus per cell was increased 37 and 90 percent, respectively." Three years later the article was published[96] in the *Annals of the New York Academy of Sciences*. If you didn't catch the significance of what you just read, it came right out and said that DDT increased the replication of poliovirus in human cells up to 90 percent.

Yet it doesn't stop there. The next chapter will begin with the mystery of amyotrophic lateral sclerosis (ALS), or Lou Gehrig's disease. There is no mystery, as pesticides, specifically organochlorine pesticides like DDT, play an important role in setting someone up for this disease.[97]

The viruses that cause polio/AFP have been around for a very long time, but then something changed, and a relatively harmless family of gut viruses started causing AFP. The "something" was the introduction of DDT and other pesticides, and viruses that had never been a problem before were able to wreak havoc in the human nervous system and replicate, buoyed by the presence of the DDT family of pesticides, but not exclusively organochlorides.

One last point here. It is known that EBV in the presence of polychlorinated biphenyl (PCB), which is an organochloride, will increase the incidence of non-Hodgkin's lymphoma (NHL) by twenty times. In Africa, there is a lymphoma called Burkitt's, the African variant of NHL that is mostly found in children, all of whom have EBV. Conventional thinking says that the combination of malaria with the EBV is what triggers this cancer. But what if we have it all wrong and it isn't the malaria that is the co-factor but the DDT exposure—just like PCBs and EBVs cause lymphoma.[98] It is something for DDT proponents to think about and factor into an evidence based policy.

## THE TOXIC SOUP WE SWIM IN

Thanks to DuPont, C-8 (perfluorooctanoic), a bio-persistent poison (never degrades in the environment), was released into the environment by the tons. DuPont had been told of the dangers of the nano-poison when the rights to C-8 were bought from 3M[99] (Minnesota Mining and Manufacturing). DuPont began a production phase-out in 2002 in response to concerns by the United States Environmental Protection Agency (EPA). It was part of Teflon, but now perfluorooctanoic is in the blood of 99.7 percent of Americans as well as in newborn human babies, breast milk, and umbilical cord blood. C-8 has been connected with rectal, kidney, and testicular cancer, and a wide assortment of birth defects. DuPont no longer uses it (at least in the United States), but the poison has been released and isn't going anywhere.

In truth, the toxic synergy of the many chemicals humans are exposed to are underappreciated and makes their removal from the environment—impossible in the case of C-8—a priority well beyond the precautionary principle.

The so-called active ingredient in any given pesticide always comes with other synergists, adjuvants, and other chemicals like solvents that are not only also toxic but sometimes far more toxic than the active ingredient. But only the active ingredient is tested because the rest of the soup is labeled inert by the manufacturer. It is a great trick played on all of us, and the regulators don't do one thing to stop this practice.

Let's use glyphosate as an example, because the situation with this pesticide is apparently reaching critical mass—everyone is starting to realize that this stuff not only doesn't biodegrade but is being used with such abandon that no one can avoid it. Glyphosate is the purported active ingredient in the most widely used pesticides worldwide. In a report released in March of 2015 and printed in the *Lancet*, the International Agency for Research on Cancer (IARC—a research arm of the World Health Organization) announced the findings of seventeen oncology experts from eleven countries. The World Health Organization has four levels of risk: known, probably, probably not, and not classifiable. Glyphosate now falls in the second level of concern.

"The widespread adoption of GMO corn and soybeans has led to an explosion in the use of glyphosate—a main ingredient in Monsanto's Roundup and Dow's Enlist Duo," said Ken Cook, president and cofounder of the Environmental Working Group. "Consumers have the right to know how their food is grown and whether their food dollars are driving up the use of a probable carcinogen."[100]

But a study published in the journal *BioMed Research International* revealed the Roundup herbicide to be 125 times more toxic than its active ingredient, glyphosate, by itself.

The paper[101] states, "Major pesticides are more toxic to human cells than their declared active principles." It demonstrates how agrichemical companies conceal the actual toxicity of the poisons they push on farmers by putting out a single ingredient as the "Trojan Horse"—the active ingredient—and from that single chemical determine an "acceptable level of harm" via the calculation of the so-called acceptable daily intake (ADI) based on the toxicological risk profile of only that single ingredient.

> Pesticides are used throughout the world as mixtures called formulations. They contain adjuvants, which are often kept confidential and are called inerts by the manufacturing companies, plus a declared active principle (AP), which is the only one tested in the longest toxicological regulatory tests performed on mammals. This allows the calculation of the acceptable daily intake (ADI)—the level of exposure that is claimed to be safe for humans over the long term—and justifies the presence of residues of these pesticides at "admissible" levels in the environment and organisms. Only the AP and one metabolite are used as markers.

Toxicity in so-called inert adjuvants was up to 10,000 times more toxic than glyphosate itself, revealing them to be a greater source for toxicity than the active ingredient.[102] This synergistic toxicity explains animal research where glyphosate products were found to be poisonous in the parts-per-trillion range (0.1 part per billion), a value that could not be explained by glyphosate itself.[103]

The researchers noted:

> Adjuvants in pesticides are generally declared as inerts, and for this rea-son they are not tested in long-term regulatory experiments. It is thus very surprising that they amplify up to 1000 times the toxicity of their APs in 100 percent of the cases where they present. In fact, the differ-ential toxicity between formulations of pesticides and their APs now appears to be a general feature of pesticides toxicology. As we have seen, the role of adjuvants is to increase AP solubility and to protect it from degradation, increasing its half-life, helping cell penetration, and thus enhancing its pesticidal activity and consequently side effects. They can even add their own toxicity.[104]

The definition of adjuvants as "inerts" is thus nonsense; even if the US Environ-mental Protection Agency has recently changed the appellation for "other ingre-dients," pesticide adjuvants should be considered as toxic "active" compounds.

According to the researchers, Roundup herbicide is an exemplary illustration of the duplicitous claims made by agrichemical corporations that the chemicals applied to our food are relatively safe and that safety is a scientific fact. It is a pseudoscience "fact" that it is safe.

The compromised public and government regulators consider Roundup one of the safest herbicides on the market. The truth is that Roundup is 125 times more toxic than glyphosate. Regardless of what we have all been brainwashed to believe, Roundup is one of the most toxic among the herbicides and insecticides tested, and it does not degrade in the environment! So, what a shock that too-big-to-fail agrichemical companies will falsify health risk assessments and delay health policy decisions at our expense so they can make money. Who would have thought that might be going on?[105] Apparently, the European Environmental Agency (EFA) thought so and published a paper, "Late lessons from early warnings," which cover a diverse range of chemical and technological innovations, and illustrates how damaging and costly is the misuse or neglect of the precautionary principle.

Until the law changes, corporations are not responsible for protecting your health with the products they sell—they are responsible only for maximizing shareholder value.

The acceptable daily intake (ADI) of glyphosate is 0.3 ppm (parts per million), but it should be less than 3 ppb (parts per billion) in the context of the Roundup, one of several glyphosate based herbicides. Glyphosate does not degrade, so it just accumulates and builds up just like DDT. The ADI is an assumption based on an assumption. No testing takes place to determine if the ADI[106] is accurate or isn't, and in the case of glyphosate, minuscule doses make for some nice endocrine disruption.

Ever wonder why so many men have "low T" (hypogonadism), girls are entering puberty at eight years of age, and women are developing breast cancer? In 2016, it was determined[107] that the endocrine-disrupting effects of all the inert ingredients and co-formulants disrupted aromatase activity, a key enzyme in the balance of sex hormones, below the toxicity threshold and 800 times lower that that used in agricultural dilution. This clearly challenges the relevance of ADI value for active ingredient exposures alone, glyphosate in this example, when the inert ingredients get a free-pass—obviously not inert.

It is never just one thing . . . and that is the whole point.

> Exposure to a single formulated pesticide must be considered as co-exposure to an AP and the adjuvants. In addition, the study of combinatorial effects of several APs together may be very secondary if the toxicity of the combinations of each AP with its adjuvants [are] neglected or unknown. Even if all these factors were known and taken into account in the regulatory process, this would not exclude an endocrine-disrupting effect below the toxicity threshold. The chronic tests of pesticides may not reflect relevant environmental exposures if only one ingredient is tested alone.

Should there be any doubt, in 2014, a report[108] came out linking glyphosate to over twenty chronic diseases:

> In the present study, US government databases were searched for GE crop data, glyphosate application data and disease epidemiological data. Correlation analyses were then performed on a total of 22 diseases in these time-series data sets. The Pearson correlation coefficients are highly significant ($< 10-5$) between glyphosate applications and hypertension (R = 0.923), stroke (R = 0.925), diabetes prevalence (R = 0.971), diabetes incidence (R = 0.935), obesity (R = 0.962), lipoprotein metabolism disorder (R = 0.973), Alzheimer's (R = 0.917), senile dementia (R = 0.994), Parkinson's (R = 0.875), multiple sclerosis (R = 0.828), autism (R = 0.989), inflammatory bowel disease (R = 0.938), intestinal infections (R = 0.974), end stage renal disease (R = 0.975), acute kidney failure (R =

0.978), cancers of the thyroid (R = 0.988), liver (R = 0.960), bladder (R = 0.981), pancreas (R = 0.918), kidney (R = 0.973) and myeloid leukaemia (R = 0.878). The Pearson correlation coefficients are highly significant (< 10–4) between the percentage of GE corn and soy planted in the US and hypertension (R = 0.961), stroke (R = 0.983), diabetes prevalence (R = 0.983), diabetes incidence (R = 0.955), obesity (R = 0.962), lipoprotein metabolism disorder (R = 0.955), Alzheimer's (R = 0.937), Parkinson's (R = 0.952), multiple sclerosis (R = 0.876), hepatitis C (R = 0.946), end stage renal disease (R = 0.958), acute kidney failure (R = 0.967), cancers of the thyroid (R = 0.938), liver (R = 0.911), bladder (R = 0.945), pancreas (R = 0.841), kidney (R = 0.940) and myeloid leukaemia (R = 0.889). The significance and strength of the correlations show that the effects of glyphosate and GE crops on human health should be further investigated.

Yep, we need "further investigation." This is the equivalent of saying, "We are not accusing anyone or anything for being dangerous or harmful. We aren't asking anyone to act. Please publish our paper. Oh, and while you are at it, could we please have another grant to study this further?"

Meanwhile, when the *New York Times* op-ed calls for the banning of glyphosate, as they did on March 25, 2015, in "Stop Making Us Guinea Pigs," you know the fix might actually be in.[109]

> We ask not whether a given chemical might cause cancer but whether we're certain that it does. Since it's unethical to test the effects of new chemicals and food additives on humans, we rely on the indirect expedient of extensive and expensive animal testing. But the job of the F.D.A. should be to guarantee a reasonable expectation of protection from danger, not to wait until people become sick before taking products off the market.

(You might have thought that government's job was to make sure products were safe before they were marketed. You'd have been wrong—Rezulin or phthalates, anyone?)

Even now, when it's clear that more research must be done to determine to what degree glyphosate may be carcinogenic, it's not clear whose responsibility it is to conduct that research. Should it be the public health agencies of other countries? Should it be independent researchers who just happen to be interested in the causes of non-Hodgkin's lymphoma, the cancer with which glyphosate is associated? We don't need better, smarter chemicals along with the few GMO crops that can tolerate them; we need fewer chemicals and a diverse genetic crop base. And it's been adequately demonstrated that crop rotation, the use of organic fertilizers, interplanting of varieties of crops, and other ecologically informed techniques commonly grouped together under the term "agroecology" can effectively reduce the use of chemicals.

Meanwhile, how about getting glyphosate and the other glyphosate based herbicides off the market until Monsanto can prove that it's safe to use? There's no reason to put the general population, and particularly the farming population, at risk for the sake of industry profits.

A class action lawsuit (Case No: BC578942)[110] was filed in Los Angeles County in May 2015 for misleading advertising. Part of it reads, "Glyphosate is linked to stomach and bowel problems, indigestion, ulcers, colitis, gluten intolerance, sleeplessness, lethargy, depression, Crohn's Disease, Celiac Disease, allergies, obesity, diabetes, infertility, liver disease, renal failure, autism, Alzheimer's, endocrine disruption, and the W.H.O. recently announced glyphosate is 'probably carcinogenic'."

The EPA classified glyphosate as a possible carcinogen in 1985. Later in 1991, when the agency changed the classification to "not carcinogenic," three scientists involved in the study refused to sign, and one wrote "do not concur." The EPA changed the classification because we now exist in a time where there is an unholy alliance between corporation and state in the United States.

## MAD AS A COW, AND WE'RE NOT GOING TO TAKE IT ANYMORE—OR ARE WE?

No discussion about glyphosate and insecticides would be complete without mentioning prions and mad cow disease. Prions are little proteins that can often be found between nerve cells in the brain. When prions malfunction, they are found to be involved in the neurodegenerative syndromes such as Creutzfeldt-Jakob disease (CJD) in humans, scrapie in sheep, chronic wasting disease in deer, and bovine spongiform encephalopathy or mad cow disease.

However, prions are not some malevolent infectious entity but normally serve an important role in neurogenesis (growth of the nervous system)[111] unless something has gone very wrong.

Prion proteins have been shown to bind copper (Cu), and Cu protects against the conversion of prions to the disease-causing form, which occurs when the presence of manganese (Mn) gets too high. Then prions bind to Mn, which induces a resistance to protein degradation by protease, a characteristic feature of prion diseases. Mn also causes the fibrils characteristic of the scrapie isoform of the protein in prion diseases.

According to Purdey,[112] the presence of mad cow disease had a direct relationship to the requirement placed on all nonorganic herds in England to the application of the organo-phthalimido-phosphorus insecticide phosmet. It was literally painted on the backs of the cattle for the control of warble fly during the 1980s. Not only does phosmet chelate Cu in the central nervous system, but it also causes oxidation of Mn to $Mn^{3+,}$ leading to its toxicity. Glyphosate chelates Cu down to much lower pH values than those at which it chelates Mn, in addition to its ability to oxidize Mn to the +3 oxidation state.

Mad cow disease is no mystery to be feared, although the deranged prions can become infectious. It was a man-made environmental disaster brought by the overuse, misuse, and abuse of pesticides—a fact that has been as well hidden as the facts surrounding pesticides causing other infectious disease outbreaks.

The very real concern here is that one could postulate that glyphosate might behave similarly to phosmet and cause prion disease under the right conditions. One can predict that glyphosate's tenacious binding to Cu will render Cu systemically unavailable, which argues for a role for glyphosate in prion diseases through Cu binding. Making Cu unavailable has implications for patients diagnosed with amyotrophic lateral sclerosis, which will be addressed.

At the hands of the agro-chemical-industrial complex, over 4.5 billion pounds of pesticides are applied each year in the United States. When Rachel Carson wrote *Silent Spring* in the early 1960s, only 400 million pounds of pesticides were used annually. Today, almost one out of two American children suffers from at least one chronic illness, and 12 million have some form of developmental disorder. The United States has the fourth highest incidence of childhood cancer in the world. Since the 1970s, there has been a 50 percent increase in childhood acute lymphocytic leukemia and a 35 percent increase in brain cancer. This new pediatric morbidity and mortality is not due to better diagnosis (a psy-op phrase the CDC is fond of using).

In July of 2016, Environmental Health Perspectives published the results of their Project TENDR: Targeting Environmental Neuro: Developmental Risks: [113]

"Children in America today are at an unacceptably high risk of developing neurodevelopmental disorders that affect the brain and nervous system including autism, attention deficit hyperactivity disorder, intellectual disabilities, and other learning and behavioral disabilities. These are complex disorders with multiple causes—genetic, social, and environmental. The contribution of toxic chemicals to these disorders can be prevented.

"The vast majority of chemicals in industrial and consumer products undergo almost no testing for developmental neurotoxicity or other health effects.

"We assert that the current system in the United States for evaluating scientific evidence and making health-based decisions about environmental chemicals is fundamentally broken."

It is interesting to note that in these occasional consensus papers critical of the United States in regulating environmental toxins to which children are exposed is counter to the position the Department of Health and Human Services takes in litigating against vaccine-injured children when their families attempt to get compensated for those injuries. It is not unlike the FDA approving THC as a prescription drug, while at the same time the DEA asserts marijuana has absolutely no redeeming medical properties.

There is an unnerving duplicity when the TENDR statement, for example, highlights the finding that there is no safe threshold exposures for lead, given it comes decades or generations too late, after millions of children are irreversibly injured. In July of 2016, the National Resource Defense Council (NRDC) announced[114] that 18 million Americans have been drinking contaminated water. EPA data was analyzed from 2015 to find that more than 5,300 water systems across the nation were in violation of the agency's Lead and Copper Rule.

Of course the system is broken when top administrators and legislators are financially beholden to industry interests: a petition submitted by Public Employees for Environmental Responsibility in March 2015 states, "USDA scientists whose work carries with it policy implications that negatively reflect upon USDA corporate stakeholder interests routinely suffer retaliation and harassment."

In 2014, more than half of food tested by the US government for pesticide residues showed detectable levels of pesticides, though almost all were within levels the government considers to be "safe," according a US Department of Agriculture report issued by the *St. Louis Post-Dispatch*.[115] "USDA said it did not test this past year [2014] for residues of glyphosate, the active ingredient in Roundup herbicide and the world's most widely used herbicide." And why would they want to test for glyphosate when "Creve Coeur–based Monsanto Co., the developer of Roundup, requested and received EPA approval for increased tolerance levels for glyphosate."[116]

That is the broken regulatory world we are subjected to—a world where the citizens depend on the government to protect them from the very businesses that have bled the government out from the inside. It is all rather misanthropically pathetic, the Golden Rule subverted to become they with the gold make the rules, write the laws, bleed out the judiciary, and buy the politicians off. But in order for our regulatory agencies to work they must maintain "scientific integrity and does not allow for harassment, censorship or suppression of findings that counter the interests of industry."[117]

But wait . . . they also bleed out the academic institutions, corrupt professional societies with their largesse, control education and the media—literally controlling which stories are published with such vast amounts of money and influence that you would find it hard to believe—and so many don't believe.

If glyphosate and Roundup, which have been in use for half a century, get removed from the market or are severely restricted, it will not be because we were being protected by the FDA, EPA, CDC, USDA, or the courts. It will have been from public pressure and a tidal wave of (real) science, but be warned . . . need I again bring up DDT and dicofol? Will that be the fate of glyphosate? Tweak it a little and rename it? But glyphosate, as dangerous as it may be, is not the most toxic component in glyphosate based herbicides—the so-called inert ingredients in Roundup that are so much more toxic than glyphosate.

In 2015, a study was published[118] titled "Agricultural insecticides threaten surface waters at the global scale" that showed that surface water contamination with pesticides exceeded the regulatory threshold levels in 66 percent of the samples tested. Samples often contained more than one pesticide, some as many as thirty. In those countries that had regulations, such as the United States, contamination was even higher than in nonregulated countries.

This is the legacy that the trillions of pounds of hazardous pesticides poured into the environment has wrought, and their role in so much illness and death is undeniable. The thing is that we let these corporations control our food supply! Why would we let this happen? Bought-and-paid-for legislators and governmental agencies have reshaped policies, regulations, and laws to benefit just a handful of corporations that now control almost every aspect of our food system from pesticide to seed. That is just insanity.

## WHAT CAN WE DO

This is the crux of the matter: we are so removed from the food we eat, so disengaged from the whole process—where and how our food is raised, and who grows it and with what. It is a reflection of our disassociation from nature as a whole.

Yelling at greedy corporations or politicians on the corporate dole will not solve this problem. Part of the solution is to become engaged in the process of the food we consume and the water we drink. Now, we can't all be farmers or all plant our own little gardens, but we can buy locally from farmers who don't use chemicals, and we can develop food and farm co-ops in which we are each members who decide what food is to be grown and how and from where, such as seed banks of non-GMO seeds. We can decide what we want to eat and to network with other co-ops and trade. In other words, we make the corporate/industrial practice of food production less and less relevant.

We have given away, in a very unconscious manner, choices about what is important to health and happiness to ruthless, nasty, and amoral entities and then scratch our collective heads about why this terrible situation has befallen us.

You can imagine that the public's interest in doing something would be great if people were immediately dropping dead on the street after eating nutritionally bankrupt and pesticide-soaked food. But it doesn't work that way, so there will need to be greater and greater efforts made to raise awareness. An informed public will be the greatest catalyst for change in this arena—hence the great efforts being made to keep us either uninformed or misinformed.

If a little girl in Napa, California, eats a handful of pesticide-soaked raspberries and immediately develops AFP, is the public told that perhaps there might be a connection? Does anyone even look at those raspberries to measure pesticide levels, and if they do will you find out about it? You can bet your sweet organic fruit you won't.

In March of 2014, I wrote a letter to California Senator Barbara Boxer via her Health Policy Advisor, Emily Katz:

> I know Senator Boxer chaired the Sub-committee on Children's Health hearing entitled, "State of Research on Potential Environmental Health Factors with Autism and Related Neurodevelopmental Disorders," back in August of 2010, and I know the bottom line from this hearing is that the rise in cases of autism is due primarily to environmental factors and that genetics only play a role in making certain children more vulnerable to toxins.
>
> The polio epidemic was also an environmental epidemic; although, no one sees it that way today. Had we learned our lesson from the poisoning of the human immune and nervous systems by a very lethal class of pesticides, which became the catalyst that caused paralysis (with or without the assistance of the virus that the whole epidemic was blamed on), I doubt we would have let the virtually uncontrollable release of so many life compromising chemicals as we have in the environment today.
>
> So good that Senator Boxer asked the CDC to look into this. I was invited once to testify at a Congressional hearing in 2004 about a very similar subject and I went down to the CDC in Atlanta in 2006 to meet with the Environmental Health Lab folks (James Pirkle and staff). Jim set me straight on how things work at the CDC. He said the Infectious Disease Division controls policy and gets all the funding, and that the Infectious Disease Division is essentially under pharmaceutical company control. I would go so far to say that pharmaceutical companies have bled out the Infectious Disease Division from the inside. This is a whole other hornet's nest I really

don't want to kick over for you here, but I was very much impressed with the concern and thoughtfulness of the Environmental Health Lab folks . . . it is just that they don't set policy nor do they call the shots, so to say, regardless of what they find and how important those findings are.

By blaming the polio epidemic of the last century on a virus and only on a virus no one had to be held accountable for the foolish use of such a lethal class of pesticides as the organochlorines (DDT, etc.) that was the real cause of the epidemic. They used to literally hose dairy herds down with DDT, and it was used everywhere, especially big cities in the USA—applied liberally and often. But if the truth about this became the acknowledged cause of so much suffering it would have heavily impacted many bottom lines.

So, my concern is . . . are we about to repeat the same mistake? It isn't enough that the neuro immune encephalopathy that is called autism has gone from 1 in 10,000 in just a couple of decades to 1 in 50 (which the CDC claims is such a big mystery to them), but now we are starting to see a return of strange paralysis cases that could be very much related to exactly what took place 60–70 years ago with the indiscriminate use of organochlorine pesticides.

We certainly don't need another hearing as much as we need swift and decisive action to limit the exposure of many nasty chemicals to which the public is exposed. But of course, there will be liability.

No, I did not receive a reply to my letter.

I blind-copied Dr. Louis Vismara (whom I had met with on a previous occasion), a retired cardiologist serving as the California Senate's full-time senior policy consultant for the California State Senate (specifically President Pro Tem Darrell Steinberg). Today he is executive director of the University Development Trust. He asked me for more details, so I wrote back to him:

Dr. Vismara:
The virus that eventually was named the polio virus, along with many other enterovirus variants, was probably a relatively harmless virus for eons—a stomach bug—until late in the 19th century. That's when a new pesticide called lead arsenate allowed the virus access to the nervous system, where it then reached the spinal cord; this combination was the trigger for the first outbreaks of the paralytic disease called poliomyelitis.

The first dozen or so outbreaks occurred in the 1890s, just as lead arsenate was invented and first used commercially. The first of those clusters was in Boston—1893 (26 cases, no deaths). In 1894, came what is widely regarded as the first major epidemic—Rutland and Proctor, Vermont (132 cases, 18 deaths). Thirty more outbreaks—from such seemingly far-flung locations as Oceana County, Michigan, and (no surprise) Napa—were reported in the United States through 1909. But the worst was in New York (1907), with 2,500 cases and a five percent mortality rate, which heralded the 1916 epidemic in the Northeast that killed 2,000 in NYC alone.

California's Napa County was undoubtedly a generous consumer of lead arsenate in grape-growing country. In fact, the San Francisco area was home to three of the first dozen outbreaks—a quarter of the total. According to the peer-reviewed journal paper, "The Spatial Dynamics of Polio,"[119] they were San Francisco and Napa, 1896 (three victims); San Joaquin Valley, 1899 (four victims); and San Francisco and vicinity, 1901 (55 victims). One fourth of the earliest clusters, were in and around San Francisco. The other clusters were in Oceana County, Michigan, (the Asparagus Capital of the World), Cherryfield, Maine (the Blueberry Capital of the World), and Boston, where there was a gypsy moth invasion in apple trees (1893).

It's hard to see how "the experts" could miss something this obvious (easy to miss something you don't want to see)—that poliomyelitis outbreaks had a toxic co-factor, which could only be lead arsenate.

The post WWII rise of DDT, as the even-deadlier replacement for lead arsenate, brought on the big polio epidemics. The heretic, Dr. Morton S. Biskind, tried to warn everyone but no one would listen to the heretic (see below).

From autism (as well as PD, ALS, MS), we've also learned that pesticides can be a risk for neurological disorders—a well-regarded study in 2007[120] found an apparent higher risk of autism in mothers who lived near farm fields in California's Central Valley, where pesticide drift is a well-known phenomenon. It called for more study, which one might have thought was a matter of urgency. After all, the first cases of autism, reported in 1943, included families with startling background exposures to the new ethylmercury compounds, including the fungicide Ceresan.

So, is this latest "polio-like" outbreak the result of another (non-polio) enterovirus? There is no evidence one way or the other yet, but toxins need to be put on table when the words "enterovirus," "San Francisco," "polio-like" and "cluster" are found in the same news stories. Remember, 3 cases of actual poliomyelitis in San Francisco in 1896 presaged 2,000 deaths in NYC just two decades later, followed by wave after worsening wave of epidemics.

I wonder how different our world would be today if the "experts" had paid attention to the evidence more than a century ago. There's still time?

In 1945, against the advice of investigators who had studied the pharmacology of the compound and found it dangerous for all forms of life, DDT was released in the United States and other countries for general use by the public as an insecticide.

Below are excerpts for Biskind's 1953 article in the *American Journal of Digestive Diseases*. Presented below are excerpts regarding polio from the article.

\*

"Since the last war there have been a number of curious changes in the incidence of certain ailments and the development of new syndromes never before observed. A most significant feature of this situation is that both man and all his domestic animals have simultaneously been affected.

"In man, the incidence of poliomyelitis has risen sharply."

\*

"It was even known by 1945 that DDT is stored in the body fat of mammals and appears in the milk. With this foreknowledge the series of catastrophic events that followed the most intensive campaign of mass poisoning in known human history, should not have surprised the experts. Yet, far from admitting a causal relationship so obvious that in any other field of biology it would be instantly accepted, virtually the entire apparatus of communication, lay and scientific alike, has been devoted to denying, concealing, suppressing, distorting and attempts to convert into its opposite, the overwhelming evidence. Libel, slander and economic boycott have not been overlooked in this campaign."

\*

"Early in 1949, as a result of studies during the previous year, the author published reports implicating DDT preparations in the syndrome widely attributed to a 'virus-X' in man, in 'X-disease' in cattle and in often fatal syndromes in dogs and cats. The relationship was promptly denied by government officials, who provided no evidence to contest the author's observations but relied solely on the prestige of government authority and sheer numbers of experts to bolster their position."

\*

"[X disease] . . . studied by the author following known exposure to DDT and related compounds and over and over again in the same patients, each time following known exposure. We have described the syndrome as follows: . . . In acute exacerbations, mild clonic convulsions involving mainly the legs, have been observed. Several young children exposed to DDT developed a limp lasting from 2 or 3 days to a week or more."

No, I did not get any further reply.

Today we know the outbreak that killed 14 and affected 1,153 people in 49 states was caused by the enterovirus EV-D68—one of more than 100 non-polio enteroviruses from which the vaccine provides no protection. In all likelihood a toxic co-factor made this breakout possible, but toxic co-factors are usually if not almost always ignored by health authorities and regulators alike. It is like trying to understand why the *Titanic* sank without considering the iceberg.

In June of 2015, a study was published that concluded,

This prospective human study links measured DDT exposure in utero to risk of breast cancer. Experimental studies are essential to confirm results and discover causal mechanisms. Findings support classification of DDT as an endocrine disruptor, a predictor of breast cancer, and a marker of high risk. . . . Many women were heavily exposed in utero during widespread DDT use in the 1960s. They are now reaching the age of heightened breast cancer risk. DDT exposure persists and use continues in Africa and Asia without clear knowledge of the consequences for the next generation.[121]

Pesticides are giving us cancer, paralysis, and other neurological disorders like AD, ALS, PD, and yet we have created a situation where it seems almost impossible to get those we have entrusted to regulate, if not protect us, to do their duty. The politics of this, the criminality of this, is beyond the scope of this book and my expertise, but clearly if we don't take action soon there will be many serious and fatal consequences.

## ZIKA

There is a real danger in blaming a lone virus for any problem. It is not unlike the obfuscation of the real problem with polio. The existence of the Zika virus has been known for many decades, but all of a sudden it has become a big problem? And a vaccine waits in the wings? Two red flags. How about the red flag that Brazil, ground zero for the crisis, uses more pesticides than perhaps any other country in the world—many of them banned in other countries. Brazil, again, is one of the countries that manufacture dicofol.

If Zika is the cause of the Brazilian microcephaly epidemic, why are there no similar epidemics in other countries also hit hard by the virus? In Brazil, the microcephaly rate soared with more than 1,500 confirmed cases. But in Colombia, a recent study of nearly 12,000 pregnant women infected with Zika found zero microcephaly cases.[122] According to a report by the New England Complex Systems Institute (NECSI), the number of missing cases in Colombia and elsewhere raises serious questions about the assumed connection between Zika and microcephaly. It is also serious that our science has been hijacked by political agendas to transfer the public's wealth—billions of dollars into vaccine R&D for an intervention that is almost certainly not needed. In "Zika and the Risk of Microcephaly"[123] researchers wrote:

> Polynesia estimated that the risk of microcephaly due to ZIKV [Zika Virus] infection in the first trimester of pregnancy was 0.95 percent (95 percent confidence interval, 0.34 to 1.91), on the basis of eight microcephaly cases identified retrospectively in a population of approximately 270,000 people with an estimated rate of ZIKV infection of 66 percent.

Not even one percent of births—hardly a global pandemic. If the CDC and the NIH want money they should study the potential triggers for microcephaly in that part of the world.

It is just so easy to blame some nasty little virus as the sole problem, and while that virus may indeed be playing a very small role, do not assume it is the main problem. It is not the truth for the poliovirus, perhaps the granddaddy of all misleading public health scams, and it is not true for Zika. Furthermore, when a disease that has been known about for more than half a century suddenly emerges . . . it makes one wonder.

If the facts don't fit the agenda, then change the facts. There is a lot of money at stake with this latest public health scare, so forget about pesticides in the drinking water and pregnant women getting whole-cell pertussis vaccines as being a cause—that isn't going to make anyone any money—in fact it will cause lawsuits and cost money. So, it is important that this be an act of nature—this evil Zika virus. In June of 2016, the *New England Journal of Medicine* published correspondence from two physicians who alerted the medical community that the CDC is recommending changing the definition of microcephaly.

In the United States there are six cases of microcephaly per 10,000 live births based on the most commonly used criterion of three SD (standard deviations) from the mean or 0.27 percent, but the CDC is now recommending any infant whose head circumference is below the 3% be diagnosed with microcephaly. When the polio vaccine came out and actually caused cases of paralysis, the definition of polio was changed to having paralysis that lasted greater than sixty days—magically thanks to the vaccine (not) cases of polio dropped dramatically—all because the definition was changed.

To justify all the money and keep the public fearful, magically the incidence of microcephaly will skyrocket if we continue to let the CDC define our reality.

## LIFE FINDS A WAY

If you haven't read the book or seen the movies, the lesson of *Jurassic Park* is that in our arrogance, we humans, blinded by both curiosity and greed, think we can splice and dice genes with no worries about the potential consequences. Ground zero for the Zika virus problem is also where the corporation Oxitec released genetically modified male mosquitoes to control the population of mosquitoes that carry several diseases. (Coincidence?) A noble endeavor to be sure, but not one without risks.[124]

The more we live in isolation from what truly supports our life here on this planet, the more we detach ourselves from nature. Generation after generation, each more detached than the last, the more we sow the seeds of our own self-destruction—it is a type of devolution. That trend needs to reverse itself. Add on to this that we have allowed ourselves to be manipulated, exploited, and experimented upon for far too long. It has never been in our interest to do so except to gain the experience of how not to live a fulfilled life.

## DETOXIFYING YOUR OWN BODY

Chapter 8 has more on the subject of detoxification, but this is a good place to mention how various toxins, pesticides, and drugs get metabolized by the body. In what is called phase I metabolism, the body (often the liver) will chemically alter a molecule it wants out of the body by making it dissolvable in water so it can leave the body. The cytochrome P450 enzyme system (CYP) is responsible for most of this activity. These enzymes are located either in the inner membrane of mitochondria or in the endoplasmic reticulum of cells. Mitochondria are often called the powerhouse of the cell because they create the fuel molecules that are used for energy in the cell. The endoplasmic reticulum is a membranous sac inside the cell.

Phase II metabolism also makes compounds water-soluble so they can be excreted, but achieves this end from a different chemical vantage point called conjugation.

Insects become resistant to pesticides, such as DDT, by having a high functioning enzyme called glutathione S-transferases (GSTs), which conjugates the reduced form of glutathione to substances for the purpose of detoxification. This would be a phase II reaction. It should be no surprise that AD patients and children with autism are known to have reduced GST activity.

Glutathione (GSH ) has multiple functions in the body, but it is an important antioxidant protecting cells from oxidative stress or damage from reactive oxygen species (ROS). ROS are produced from the metabolism of oxygen, but stress and toxins can increase ROS that can facilitate cell damage—think hydrogen peroxide levels getting too high in your cells.

There is also a phase III metabolic pathway in which, following phase II, certain molecules may need further modification before they can be excreted.

Diet influences both phase I and II systems. Protein deficiency decreases CYP metabolism while high protein diets increase it. Conversely, a high carb diet will decrease CYP activity. Micronutrients, such as vitamins A, $B_2$ (riboflavin), $B_3$ (niacin), folate, C, E, iron, calcium, copper, zinc, magnesium, and selenium need to be at optimal levels to have efficient phase I activity. St. John's Wort (hypericum) is a phase I inducer, but as a precaution, taking any given medicinal herb is not compatible with everyone, especially on a long-term basis.

I consider hypericum to be a medicinal herb, which means it needs to be taken with the appropriate precautions and instructions. A medicinal food or plant, like garlic, can be taken every day in various amounts without any special precautions or instructions (unless you are allergic to garlic).

The plants that belong to the *Brassica* family, such as cabbage, broccoli, and brussels sprouts, are medicinal foods because they contain indole-3-carbinol, which stimulates both phase I and phase II systems. Oranges and tangerines (as well as the seeds of caraway and dill) contain limonene, a terpene that has been found to be a strong inducer of both phase I and phase II enzymes. Limonene takes its name from the lemon and it is responsible for the smell of citrus fruits—especially concentrated in the rind. Note: Naringenin (the principal flavonoid in grapefruit) inhibits CYP activity.

GSH conjugation is one of six phase II detoxification pathways. Reduced glutathione (GSH for GST conjugation) depends on adequate dietary sulfur-containing amino acids (methionine and cysteine), vitamin $B_6$ such as pyridoxal-5-phosphate (P5P) for the conversion of methionine to cysteine, as well as vitamins $B_2$ and $B_3$ for the activity of glutathione reductase, which recycles oxidized GSH.

S-adenosylmethionine (SAM-e), a component of the methylation cycle, another phase II pathway, stimulates GST activity by mediating GSH efficacy. The more SAM-e one consumes, the more GST is stimulated. Having said that, SAM-e should be considered a medicinal nutrient, not a medicinal food. Taking mass quantities of SAM-e could cause some individuals untoward problems, such as anxiety, headaches, and insomnia. It is always best to seek the counsel of an experienced naturopath, functional nutritionist, or functional physician if you are inclined to take large quantities of anything.

Green tea, or epigallocatechin gallate (EGCG), can increase CYP activity and increase phase II activity (GST) as well. Garlic will increase GST activity. Resveratrol, curcumin, cinnamon, α-Lipoic acid (ALA), alpha tocopherol, lycopene, gingko biloba, chalcone, capsaicin, hydroxytyrosol from olives, chlorophyllin[125], and many others will all increase phase II activity.

Some supplements are more potent than others, such as glucoraphanin from broccoli (also known as sulforaphane glucosinolate or "sgs"), and strongly bring up GSH levels.

This quick start list might help you organize the above information, but as confusing as it may all seem, you have to understand why you might want to take a particular supplement if you are actually going to follow through and take it. Detoxification from pesticides does not happen overnight, and it can require swallowing a lot of supplements for a very long time. I have put certain doses next to these supplements, but certain individuals are more sensitive than others and could tolerate or need much higher doses depending on their circumstance.

- N-acetyl cysteine: suggested dose of 600 mg one to three times daily. (Note: Always start low and work yourself up to full doses)
- Green tea extract; standardized EGCG: 800 mg to 3 grams daily. (Note: Get the no-caffeine version)
- Quercetin: 250–500 mg daily
- B vitamin complex: follow label instructions (Note: If you have a double MTHFR mutation, you don't want folic acid—you want folinic acid)
- Magnesium: 300–600 mg daily. (Note: Start low in case your bowels are very sensitive)
- Broccoli sprout or seed extract; glucoraphanin 400 mg once or twice daily, with meals
- I3C (Indole-3-carbinol): 80–160 mg daily
- SAM-e: 400 mg two to three times daily
- Milk thistle extract; standardized to silymarin and silibinins: 750 mg daily
- α-Lipoic acid (ALA): 200–500 mg daily
- Calcium-D-glucarate: 140–300 mg daily
- Resveratrol: 250 mg daily
- Curcumin: 400 mg to 4 grams, daily with meals
- Chlorophyllin: 100 mg three times per day with food
- Artichoke extract: 500 mg daily

# 3

# Human Colony Collapse Disorder (Thanks for all the Fish!)[88]

*"I regard consensus science as an extremely pernicious development that ought to be stopped cold in its tracks. Historically, the claim of consensus has been the first refuge of scoundrels; it is a way to avoid debate by claiming that the matter is already settled. Whenever you hear the consensus of scientists agrees on something or other, reach for your wallet, because you're being had."*

*"There is no such thing as consensus science. If it's consensus, it isn't science. If it's science, it isn't consensus. Period."*[126]

—Michael Crichton

In the first chapter on Lyme it became clear that, with all the earmarks of a plague, the powers that be are willing to let millions go underdiagnosed and undertreated in some quasi-suicidal alliance between academia, the CDC, and big pharmaceutical companies. In the second chapter, it was revealed that we have allowed a few to both poison the food supply and control it with no functional oversight—at a considerable cost to the rest of us. This chapter asks the question, do we really want to exterminate ourselves so that a few can sell their wares? Follow this White Rabbit down the hole, and we are face-to-face with Human Colony Collapse Disorder, all because we have unconsciously trusted those who never deserved that trust.

What is taking place with bees and their colony collapse disorder (CCD) is now taking place in humans. The circumstance is a little different. For us, it is a collection of "incurable" diseases that are just one big "mystery." But what is taking place now in humanity is not a collection of crop circles—an actual mystery. What is taking place now in humanity is a grand poisoning.

But first, here is a tale with a happy ending. In 2005, Barry J. Marshall, AC, FRACP, FRS, FAA, and DSc (honorary), received the Nobel Prize in Physiology or Medicine (along with Robin Warren, his long-time collaborator) "for their discovery of the bacterium *Helicobacter pylori* and its role in gastritis and peptic ulcer disease."[127] For those of you who were around watching TV in the '70s and '80s, antacid commercials were run just about every ten seconds on some station. It was big business, because a lot of people had peptic ulcer disease, and the medical community could only tell people to take antacids for it.

Convinced that a strange spiral bacteria Marshall cultured was the cause of so much gastritis and peptic ulcer disease, he tried to create an animal model but failed, so in 1984 he drank a vat of *H. pylori,* and in days he had the answer he was looking for. How he avoided being assassinated by all those antacid manufacturers is almost a mystery, but it may have had something to do with the fact this all took place in Australia and providence protected him. The antacid commercials disappeared almost overnight when conventional medicine could not doubt the science these two men brought to light.

The above story, while true, is not what usually takes place. The story of Marshall, Warren, and *H. pylori* is the exception to the rule.

The rule is that if a pharmaceutical corporation is not positioned to make gobs of money on a new drug related to a discovery, the information just languishes in a journal and is never translated into the clinical practice of medicine, where illness is treated in the "real" world.

You can be a very ethical pharmaceutical company, and if there is one out there, and there probably is, you can bet it is what I call a one-drug-wonder company—a relatively small enterprise that only has one drug to sell for the most part. The expense to get approval or add another indication with the FDA for a drug, depending on what that indication is for, can run into the hundreds of millions of dollars. Now that is a lot of money, so if you or I came up with the cure of something and it was patentable, just where would that kind of money come from? Or what if an old drug that is out of patent was found to cure this or that? A product without profit is difficult to invest in for reasons obvious.

The system we have certainly is not geared to assist in innovation or what might be best for patients. It is all a business, a for-profit business geared to sell something, whether that something is the best or the worst, but sell it must. Therefore, the system is as broken as much as the agencies that regulate healthcare and drugs.

Before we leave the subject of *H. pylori,* note that there is an alternative to antibiotics. A tree resin called mastic gum (*Pistacia lentiscus*) has been found to be almost as effective as antibiotics in treating the bacterial infection that causes peptic ulcers. The published studies that do not support its use are usually methodologically flawed, such as a study group that was too small (*N*).[128]

It is important to point out that there are usually alternatives to the standard or accepted methods of treating various disease states. Some are better or more efficient than others. Greed is not reserved for pharmaceutical companies. Nevertheless, wouldn't it be nice if we had access to all the options so we could make informed decisions?

Sharyl Attkisson, an award-winning journalist, stated on February 6, 2015, "There are widespread efforts to create what I call a false reality to engulf you when you're exposed to most any forms of media." The idea is to give the impression there's widespread support for or against an agenda when there may not really be. Those behind the efforts to sway your opinion, sometimes using bullying tactics, are special interests that want to make debates seem ended, science seem settled, and you feel like an outlier—when none of those things is actually the case.

We would have more options if we stopped letting ourselves be so easily manipulated. Few have any concept of how little respect the would-be despots among us and their henchmen have for the public. Fake grassroots efforts are paraded in front of us that put the pro-tobacco campaigns of old to shame. Astroturf (fake grassroots) organizations are created by PR agencies—fake blogs, fake stories, fake news feeds, and demonizing campaigns to personally discredit truth tellers and truth seekers. Those of their ilk have us so well trained that if someone brings up a topic they don't want the public to discuss or think about, they have us quasi-hypnotized to shut down our thinking processes.

Using the 9/11 attacks to illustrate the process of how to turn off critical thinking, let's assume well over the majority of Americans, and Canadians for that matter, don't believe the official story. That is what the pollsters tell us depending on the year the poll was taken or by whom, there may be only 10 percent of Americans who still believe the government is telling the truth about 9/11. If you think those polls went unnoticed, think again. They in part explain the frantic drive toward control and surveillance—a tyranny hoping to birth itself as fast as possible—before the inertia of the public rises up and the truth comes to the fore. The media is fully complicit in this apparent false flag event. If there is any doubt about how controlled the media is, look out at an almost complete blackout on what Fukushima is doing to sea life in the Pacific.

Sometimes it is simply too uncomfortable to embrace the realization of what humans have done to each other. It is psychologically too stressful to acknowledge that so many scumbags walk among us, so it doesn't take too much encouragement to shut down our critical thinking when confronted with information that questions the official pronouncement of "reality." This is nothing new, and there are many examples.[129]

## NEURODEGENERATIVE DISEASE IS THE FLAGSHIP SYMPTOM OF HUMAN COLONY COLLAPSE DISORDER

If there ever was a mysterious incurable disease, amyotrophic lateral sclerosis (ALS) would seem to fit the bill. It is a disease in which motor neurons are crippled, and its hallmark is progressive muscle weakness without notable sensory loss (touch sensation). The end-stage disease may be in the spinal cord, but its cause is not in the spinal cord. Approximately 20,000 people in the United States have ALS, and 5,000 people are diagnosed with ALS each year. ALS is common worldwide, affecting people of all races and ethnic backgrounds. The average age of onset of ALS is between forty and sixty years of age, but ALS can strike both younger and older men and women. About 5 percent to 10 percent of cases are familial (genetic), and there are several genes involved. But there is no question that ALS is an infectious/environmental illness, and familial cases may just be exquisitely sensitive to the triggers.

Nothing makes the point stronger for ALS being an environmental illness than noting that military veterans are 50 percent to 60 percent more likely to develop ALS and die from the disease than those with no history of military service, regardless of their branch of service, the era in which they served, and whether they served during times of war or peace.[130] Gulf War veterans are twice as likely as other veterans to develop ALS, but it is all a big "mystery." Health authorities like that word. It is a safe bet that when you hear the word "mystery" in this context, it is almost always an environmental/infectious disease issue.

## MEET HTLV, HUMAN ENDOGENOUS RETROVIRUS-K AND TDP-43

The Wikipedia page for HTLV begins with "Human T-cell lymphotropic virus type 1 or human T-lymphotropic virus type 1 (HTLV-I), also called the adult T-cell lymphoma virus type 1, is a retrovirus of the human T-lymphotropic virus (HTLV) family that has been implicated in several kinds of diseases."

The interesting thing is HTLV causes HTLV-I-associated myelopathy (HAM) and tropical spastic paraparesis (TSP). Less than 4 percent of HTLV victims will go on to develop HAM/TSP, but the point is HAM/TSP causes symptoms very similar to ALS, but that is not the whole story.

Present in the human genome lie a great many viral DNA sequences and most remain silent. However, under certain conditions such as pesticide exposure, these viruses can get expressed. Li et al.[131] now report that one such virus, human endogenous retrovirus-K, is expressed in neurons of a subpopulation of patients with ALS. The envelope protein of this virus causes degeneration of neurons, and transgenic animals expressing this protein develop an ALS-like syndrome caused by nucleolar dysfunction in motor neurons. Reactivation of the virus is regulated by the transcription factor TDP-43. Thus, therapeutic approaches against this virus could potentially alter the course of the disease.

Today a pharmaceutical company is in clinical trials with a neurotrophic factor called GM604:

> A number of rugby athletes who are recently being treated by GM604 have been exposed to pesticides applied to playing fields. Some of them have the habit of licking their fingers to get a better grip of the ball. In the absence of functioning TDP-43, toxic pesticides and harmful chemicals as random segments of RNA may inject themselves during protein formation to create faulty/misfolded proteins within the cell causing the neural cells to die. GM604 can modulate TDP-43 and stop the formation of random misfolded proteins by toxins.[132]

The point is not about how helpful GM604 will be but the connection back to pesticides as the ultimate underlying trigger in so many neurodegenerative diseases. We can focus on this virus or that virus as we need to because treating them may help patients, but if it were not for the pesticides, the problem wouldn't exist.

## ENVIRONMENTAL LAW HAS BECOME PABULUM IN THE HANDS OF POLITICIZED AGENCIES

It should come as no surprise that a meta-analysis found that ALS risk is associated with use of pesticides, particularly the organochlorine pesticides that were so prominently featured in the last chapter on dementia.[133] Now, it is never one thing, but at the risk of sounding like a broken record, it should be becoming quite clear that we are poisoning ourselves with pesticides and they are a hindrance to advanced life on this planet, even humans. (It's difficult to put humans in the category of "advanced" life given how apparently stupid we are if we allow a few to destroy life on this planet.)

The second most common neurodegenerative disease after Alzheimer's is Parkinson's disease (PD). Neuronal protein accumulations called Lewy bodies[134]—a pathologic feature of Parkinson's—are also found in the brains of Alzheimer's patients; PD-afflicted brains often contain the amyloid protein aggregates common to Alzheimer's.

There is an enzyme called cytochrome P450 2D6 (CYP2D6) that metabolizes and eliminates 25 percent of prescription drugs. If you are a poor metabolizer because your CYP2D6 has a genetic polymorphism, then that doubles the risk of developing PD.[135]

Paraquat exposure increases the risk of developing PD 2.5-fold, and many pesticides are associated with increased Parkinson's risk by inhibiting an enzyme called ALDH, which also detoxifies the dopamine metabolite DOPAL. When the enzyme isn't working properly, DOPAL builds up in neurons and may explain the loss of dopaminergic neurons in Parkinson's.

## COPPER AND ALS

A dismutation of the copper-zinc superoxide-dismutase (CuZnSOD1) gene occurs in about 20 percent of hereditary ALS. SOD (superoxide dismutases) are enzymes that break up the toxic superoxide ($O2^-$) radical into either ordinary molecular oxygen ($O_2$) or hydrogen peroxide ($H_2O_2$). Obviously, a less-than-stellar ability to rid the body of these dangerous free radicals could really impact our physiological integrity when exposed to poisons that increase the need to detoxify free radicals. There is great hope PET-imaging agent (tracer) CuATSM will be therapeutic in familial if not all ALS patients as it seems to get the copper (Cu) into the enzyme and correct the problem with the enzyme.

There is just something about pesticides and copper that is not fully understood—remember, copper protects prions from turning into mutated forms.

The latest research shows that AD, PD, and ALS share a common, or at least overlapping, pathologic mechanism(s).[136] This implies that AD, PD, and ALS are essentially the same disease with a slight variation on a theme. The theme is pesticide poisoning, and there is a synergistic[137] effect of heavy metals (think aluminum and mercury) with pesticides in the creation of the misfolded α-synuclein fibrils. Pesticides directly accelerate the rate of α-synuclein fibril formation.[138]Add onto this various opportunistic biological issues, such as the neurospirochetosis that are present in 90 percent of the brains of AD patients, and you can see that AD, ALS, and PD is more than about just one thing. Pesticides affect the microglial[139] cells in the brain, and these specialized white blood cells simply don't do their jobs helping to clean up and protect the way they are supposed to do. I know there is a pharmaceutical company, even now, trying to bring to the market a drug that will revive microglial function. The company may even eventually claim it as a quasi-cure for some of these disorders, but as always this would sidestep what poisoned the microglia in the first place.

But no one needs a drug to do this when curcumin already has them all beat, which is why if one has a neurodegenerative disorder, large amounts of curcumin can be extremely helpful.[140] Add in vitamin $D_3$ and the curcumin deconstructs the infamous amyloid plaques found in AD.[141]

## IF WE CANNOT ADDRESS THE PESTICIDE ISSUE, WE ARE SIMPLY DOOMING OURSELVES

Opportunistic infections are usually not isolated events, as there may be several going at it at the same time. One of the families of organisms is called mycoplasma.[142] These are bacteria without cell walls. And when other chronic disease (poisonings?) states, such as Gulf War syndrome, chronic fatigue syndrome (myalgic encephalomyelitis), and rheumatoid arthritis (RA), are treated by antibiotics,[143] (often requiring six rounds of those six-week courses), many patients clinically improve.[144]

It bears repeating: RA is not the poster child of autoimmunity that is drilled into medical students and everyone else. It is most often an infection with a mycoplasma organism. There is obviously an immune reaction—that is not in question—but the trigger is not some mysterious allergy to self: it is due to an infection. And while some in the know may merely call the infection a "cofactor," it is no different from calling the *Streptococcus* bacterium ("strep") a cofactor in a strep throat.

How long has the medical literature been publishing on the connection between mycoplasma and RA? There are studies that go back to the last century,[145] some of which go back fifty years, which in the world of medicine is a very, very long time. Financial conflicts of interest can have a very pernicious influence on progress in the medical field. Those financially conflicted will fund studies meant to cast doubt by not finding the organism or using techniques guaranteed not to find the organism, either intentionally or unintentionally.

## "IT'S NOT MY JOB"

It is not the job of a pharmaceutical company to educate the medical community about the truth of a particular medical condition. Their job, as previously explained, is to sell their product, but one could assume that if anyone knows the true nature of a medical problem, it will be those whose business it is to know. Pharmaceutical company legal departments make sure they say something like "If you have a serious infection, this drug should not be used; ask your doctor." That line is repeated many times in direct consumer advertisements to the public. But the irony is asking a physician if you have a serious chronic infection is a classic catch-22 when few know where to look—or correctly interpret the results should they look.

There are physicians who will completely deny the existence of some of these diseases because they don't know enough to do their job or are too self-important to admit to themselves how they are up to their eyeballs in their own intellectual hubris. If that sounds arrogant, callous, and perhaps even self-aggrandizing, if you suffer from a chronic illness you probably have run into some of these individuals.

Even when you can document for a patient the presence of an organism's DNA in a lab test, the so-called infectious disease authorities may dismiss it. The resistance that many have in medicine to a reality that does not jibe with their current understanding is a combination of being enmeshed in a pattern of thinking in which an ability to understand facts or/and an inability to integrate new facts unless they come packaged in a certain way (like a new drug being marketed). It is difficult for someone who believes they know everything to consider that they may have missed something or misled patients for years. Coming to terms with that takes a level of character that seemingly is not that accessible to many in the academic medical community—if you think you are a Big Kahuna, you often have an ego to match.

Sometimes I think it wouldn't be such a bad idea to have a medical Big Kahuna who is 100 percent free of conflict of interest and beyond reproach and who can issue medical proclamations regardless of whose toes might be stepped on in the process. Just announce what is in the best interest of patients without fear of reprisal. A medical pharaoh!

My sense is that the time of the pharaohs and Big Kahunas is past, and the collective must become their own parent, so to speak, and both understand and take responsibility in this arena, because if this does not happen, human colony collapse is inevitable.

Most of us enjoyed a childhood where we knew our parents were looking after our best interests, and it is natural to transfer those paternal feelings to institutions and governmental agencies when we become adults, but the sad truth is that is not the way things are working. When we give our blind trust to conflicted and compromised organizations, then the tendency has been that they will take advantage of that trust. Power and money corrupt, which should not come as a surprise.

For example, the official US government (USDA) position on bee colony collapse disorder (CCD) is that there is no consistent pattern on pesticide use and CCD, and while they are willing to concede that pesticides may have a role to play, CCD is still all a mystery. And you don't have to regulate or impose legislative restrictions when no one has all the answers—doesn't that sound so reasonable and familiar?

This playbook gets used over and over because the necromancers who want to control our lives know it has worked before, and they do have to control their deluded minions, so they need playbooks. This is what happens when industry imposes a culture of undue influence on a system that was mandated to protect and serve, a system almost completely bled out by industry insiders, lobbyists, who then write legislation and get financially compromised legislators to pass laws that make it easier for the industry to continue to do what they do—selling their stuff no matter how deleterious it is. Control academia, control regulatory agencies, control the regulations, control the law, control the courts, and then control the press. It has become that pernicious. Silence critics by ignoring them, marginalizing them, and discrediting them—if necessary, destroy anyone naive enough to speak the truth.

While there are those who would like to think humankind is independent from the environment, there is no separation between man and his environment, and CCD could herald *human* colony collapse disorder. We have gotten ourselves in a situation where it is now by our own individual and collective free will and choice to do nothing or take action. If the Harvard School of Public Health (HSPH) comes out and says that pesticides are the cause of CCD,[146] and that isn't enough to change the way we approach the pesticide problem, then whom do we have to blame but ourselves? Sure, there are always critics: "The sample size was too small, the studies aren't published in the correct journals (controlled by industry), the author picks his toes in Poughkeepsie," and so on. Creating doubt, creating plausible deniability, and creating faux theories give a compromised and corrupt system a way to avoid being held responsible. The system is broken.

This is the science: "We conclude that when honey bees were exposed to either imidacloprid or clothianidin . . . six of twelve previously healthy neonicotinoid-treated colonies died and all progressed to exhibit CCD symptoms during the winter months."[147]

The agribusiness industry will insist on how complex and uncertain things are and how policy makers shouldn't make decisions under pressure (unless the pressure is coming from agribusiness). They will say anything to get their way, but eventually you can't deny the obvious if you get hit over the head with it, as seems too often to be the case.

Finally, in early 2016, the EPA in a "preliminary risk assessment" was willing to concede that maybe neonicotinoids[148] could be causing CCD and they will take another look at it (twenty-two years after approving imidacloprid).

In Europe three neonicotinoid insecticides have now been banned, but the precautionary ban applies only to three of seven neonicotinoids and only for use with "crops attractive to bees." So it does not take into account the impacts of neonicotinoids on aquatic invertebrate species, birds, or insects, which are also major areas of concern. Neither does the ban cover new neonicotinoid insecticides. Agrichemical companies are always trying to figure out a way around restrictions and bans, as DDT/dicofol discussed in the previous chapter illustrated.

By the end of May 2015, the EPA proposed creating temporary pesticide-free zones when certain plants are in bloom around bees that are trucked in, such as in what takes place in almond groves. But the EPA's position is that pesticides are indispensable, and we just need to create a better way to live with them. This kind of compromise is emblematic of a disconnect that still continues. Pesticides are not indispensable in agriculture—there are always alternatives, and alternatives that do not harm us or the environment.

Also, bees sent to almond groves, for example, don't all stay in those groves. They go outside to forage, and if they run into flowers on plants whose seeds were soaked in the nicotinoids, then the nectar of the flowers is contaminated, and it doesn't take much to poison the hive. When you have the same companies controlling seed and pesticide, you have the problem we have today.

Even when officials are moved to action, this disconnect is so severe that the government will propose an almost worthless solution. The US Fish and Wildlife Service will now be spending a mere $2 million to help bring back the monarch butterfly. Their dwindling numbers are blamed on decrease in milkweed habitat and farms. Nothing is said to the public about what is going on at farms—Roundup-ready crops and the massive amounts of glyphosate used on them. It was certainly mentioned as the main problem in the report by the Center for Food Safety.[149] Planting more milkweed is not going to solve this problem. This is not about loss of habitat; this is about a mass poisoning.

One more example: "Developmental pesticide exposure reproduces features of attention deficit hyperactivity disorder"[150] was an article published in 2015. It reveals that if pyrethroid pesticide metabolites were found in children's urine, they were twice as likely to be diagnosed with ADHD. From polio to ADHD and everything in between—one pesticide or another is always in the mix. But it is never one thing.

In June 2015, a study was published in the journal *PLOS ONE*.[151] It states, "Aluminum is the most significant environmental contaminant of recent times." The abstract of the article starts out,

> Herein we have measured the content of aluminum in bumblebee pupae taken from naturally foraging colonies in the UK. . . . While no other statistically significant relationships were found relating aluminum to bee or colony health, the actual content of aluminum in pupae are extremely high and demonstrate significant exposure to aluminum. Bees rely heavily on cognitive function and aluminum is a known neurotoxin with links, for example, to Alzheimer's disease in humans. The significant contamination of bumblebee pupae by aluminum raises the intriguing spectre of cognitive dysfunction playing a role in their population decline.

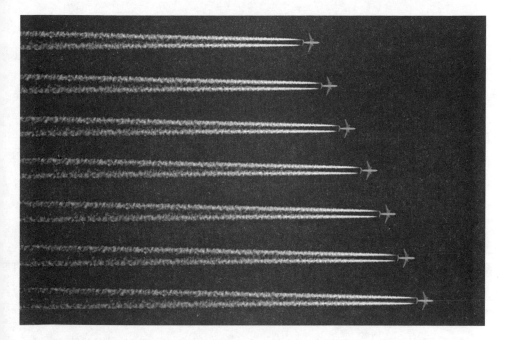

Gee . . . you think?

But where is the aluminum coming from?

For more than a decade, the United States, and now all NATO countries, have been subjected to a clandestine aerosol assault known as Stratospheric Aerosol Geoengineering. The toxic brew that is sprayed isn't always the same, but it is reported to include barium, nano aluminum-coated fiberglass (known as CHAFF), radioactive thorium, cadmium, chromium, nickel, desiccated blood, mold spores, yellow fungal mycotoxins, and ethylene dibromide. Occasionally, local weather reports will talk about them because they sometimes show up on Doppler radar, and they will say they are not clouds or a front. Beyond that there is a complete news blackout.

It would be nice if it were possible to put a happy face on these revelations, but how does one put a happy face on the fact that we are allowing a few greedy corporations and powerful control freaks that have bled out the government to make money at our expense and at the expense of a great deal of life on this planet? Do you write your congressman? Your congressman will call for a congressional hearing, and a parade of other government officials who are all on the take and paid-off experts will blabber on about the science not being completely in, mysterious factors at work, or how they are checking in on all of this and have been for some time. The hearing ends and nothing gets accomplished.

## THE BOTTOM LINE

Just because we have pesticides doesn't mean they should be used or used in the way they are currently.

## A COCONUTTY TREATMENT

Mitochondria are the little organelles in each of our cells that act as energy generators. They take oxygen and glucose and convert them into the gasoline our cells run on—ATP. Many of us learned that in high school biology. There is no question that there is mitochondrial dysfunction in the nerve cells of patients with neurodegenerative disorders, such as ALS, PD, and AD.

Perhaps you have heard about how coconut oil seems to benefit people who suffer from this group of disorders, and there is a very simple explanation as to why we know it helps: the stories are true.[152] It is the caprylic acid in coconut oil, which accounts for about 9 percent of the oil that is responsible for the therapeutic benefit. So strong is the evidence that caprylic acid benefits those with the disorders that the FDA approved a medicinal food called caprylidene (trade name Axona).

Caprylic acid is a medium-chain (C8) triglyceride that is metabolized to ketone bodies, and the mitochondria are designed to use ketone bodies as fuel if they either can't get the needed amount of glucose (because one is starving/fasting or just not eating), or the glucose is there but for some reason isn't being brought into the cell. It is here that these ketone bodies provide alternative energy source for neurons and thus compensate for mitochondrial dysfunction. If there is no mitochondrial dysfunction, there is no benefit from caprylic acid.

Consuming caprylic acid is a backdoor way to offset impairment of mitochondrial function, and thus energy metabolism, regardless of what is causing that impairment. This fat does cross the blood-brain barrier and has been found to have anticonvulsant (antiseizure) properties, which is no surprise given that convulsions are caused for the most part by mitochondrial dysfunction. Anything that preserves a neuron's ability to function has a neuroprotective effect.[153]

For the caprylic acid to work, the consumption of caprylic triglycerides should account for at least 10 percent of the daily calories in the diet. Coconut oil has about 100 calories per tablespoon (15 cc). If we assume that pure caprylic triglycerides have that calorie count as well, one would need to consume one tablespoon worth of caprylic triglycerides for every 900 calories in the diet. If one were just using coconut oil itself, where the caprylic acid is only 10 percent by weight, then we are looking at 150 cc of coconut oil per every 900 calories in the diet, or 5 ounces of coconut oil.

One does not need coconut oil or caprylic triglycerides to create ketones, but it seems easier than going on a ketogenic diet.[154]

Pure caprylic triglycerdies can be purchased (as of the writing of this book) at a wholesale supplier to the cosmetic trade[155] at about the same cost as coconut oil itself. If increasing ketone levels works for a patient with AD/PD/ALS,[156] it might be of benefit to supplement with the B vitamin, panothenic acid (vitamin B$_5$), L-carnitine, and CoQ-10 to see if there is additional benefit. Now, this is not a cure, and it does not remove toxins, but where there is energy there is hope, and certainly worth a try as it is completely benign.

A word on Parkinson's disease: assuming one does not have Lyme or Parkinsonism from a toxic exposure, such as carbon monoxide, it is worth a trial of 4-PAS or 5-ASA, which will selectively chelate manganese (Mn) from the human body. Mn is an essential trace element but can be absorbed or ingested in toxic forms and in excess. Exposure can be from gasoline to well water.

If the 4-PAS or 5-ASA changes symptoms, this is about Mn toxicity issues.[157] Glutathione is not a specific detoxification agent for just Mn, but a large dose will help remove some of it.

Mesalazine, also known as mesalamine, is 5-aminosalicylic acid (5-ASA), and like 4-PAS is considered by conventional medicine to be anti-inflammatory because it helps treat inflammatory bowel disease. It is the active part of the antibiotic sulfasalazine, which is used to treat Crohn's disease. This leads us into the next chapter, where we find out conventional medicine has it wrong again.

# 4

# Inflammatory Bowel Disease, or what a pile of . . .

*"The US medical system kills 225,000 people every year. That's 2.25 million killings per decade."*

—Dr. Barbara Starfield, *JAMA*, July 26, 2000,
"Is US Health Really the Best in the World?"

To put Dr. Starfield's estimate of the number of people killed annually by the US medical system—225,000—into perspective, it is about half of what the American death toll on Normandy Beach (WWII) would be every year, and seventy-five times what the 9/11 death toll would be every year. And I would say that is a very conservative number. Yet it doesn't make the news.

I started dating my first girlfriend when I was seventeen. She had already had loops of bowel surgically removed because she had this disease called Crohn's disease (CD), which is one of the inflammatory bowel diseases (such as "autoimmune" proctitis). It causes chronic diarrhea, abdominal pain, and weight loss. Fast-forward a decade later when I was on rounds as a young pediatric resident asking the chairman of the department, "Why are we were treating that teenager with CD with sulfasalazine when this was an autoimmune disease?" Dr. Ben Kagan told me we were using antibiotics because they seemed to have anti-inflammatory properties that benefited CD. Anti-inflammatory properties or not, they were at least partially effective with lowering the count of infectious organisms that are the cause of CD.

Thirty years later, and despite clinical trials being completed showing how a combination of several antimicrobial agents did in the organism at the root cause of most cases of CD, ulcerative colitis (UC), "autoimmune" proctitis, and irritable (inflammatory) bowel syndrome/disorder (IBS/IBD), the rest of the medical community is still back there on rounds with Dr. Kagan. Pull any physician aside and ask them to tell you about *Mycobacterium avium,* and they will shrug their collective shoulders unless they work with HIV patients.

A bacterium known as *Mycobacterium avium paratuberculosis* (MAP)[158] is found in the gut of cattle and other ruminants suffering from a disease called Johne's, as well as in the intestines of many Crohn's and ulcerative colitis patients. At least five million people suffer from IBD globally.

So engrained is the autoimmune theory that almost any disease we don't have a full understanding of as to why it exists must be an autoimmune disease. It would take the full marketing power of a pharmaceutical company to change the way physicians understand these bowel disorders. Fortunately there is a pharmaceutical company that has put several of these agents together in one pill so they can get a unique patent on drugs that are long off-patent. They are currently doing clinical trials with this new combo pill, but until they are ready to market the pill, physicians aren't going to know about it unless they go out of their way to flesh out the press releases of pharmaceutical companies[159] or actually read the relevant medical literature themselves. If you think reading the relevant medical literature is part of a physician's job, think again.

The closest thing to a real autoimmune disease is caused by the side effects from vaccine (remember the LYMErix vaccine from chapter 1). That would make it an iatrogenic (physician-caused) illness more than an autoimmune one. But some of the ingredients in vaccines are proteins and other molecules that exist in the human body or very closely resemble them, so when the body develops an immune response to the vaccine, it goes after those antigens wherever they exist in the body. For example, if they exist in your brain, you will start attacking your own brain, but it will be a big mystery to your physician, who doesn't read either the package inserts of the vaccine or the medical literature documenting all the cases of untoward vaccine reactions. Maybe they watch C-Span so they can hear some public health officials from the CDC prevaricate to Congress when asked if vaccines cause brain damage.

The prevalence of MAP infection in Western European and North American dairy herds can be well over half the herd.[160] Infected animals shed MAP in their milk, and humans consume the milk. MAP in CD, UC, and IBD is present in a protease-resistant, nonbacillary form. It can evade immune recognition and likely causes immune dysregulation—a fancy way to name when the immune system spazzes out. This organism, which is more robust than the mycobacterium that causes tuberculosis, is found in hot tubs and showerheads, but one is more likely to get a lung infection than a gut infection from those sources—always a good idea to regularly spray down certain areas of the bathroom and fixtures with hydrogen peroxide.

Yet again we have another group of diseases caused by an infectious agent allowed to run amok because no one in authority seems to care about its presence, even though its presence is another public health emergency. But who is in authority to declare this emergency?

No one (with any integrity or smarts) apparently.

How does one get something to be a public health emergency? I am sure the residents of Flint were asking each other that question. But let a few cases of measles[161] show up in almost all vaccinated individuals, and some people are ready to burn their non-vaccinating neighbors at the stake. Do you know what the actual death rate is for measles?

The CDC might tell you it is 1 in 800, but that might be the rate only if you include all third world countries. In the United States, between 2004 and 2015, no one died of measles. The twelve-year mortality for CD, IBD, and UC is 1 in 4.5.[162] Where is the outcry?

The hype around the Disneyland measles outbreak was pure manipulation by a pharmaceutical company, the CDC, and the American Legislative Exchange Council (ALEC) to increase vaccine sales by removing parental rights.[163] You might want to read the lawsuits against Merck for violation of the False Claims Act for producing a worthless and dangerous vaccine. The revelations deal with what lengths vaccine manufacturers will go to control the market, have no liability nor care if their vaccines actually work or not.

## TREATING IBD

So, how does one treat CD, IBD, autoimmune proctitis, and UC when they are "idiopathic" (of unknown cause)?

I am going to put in another good word for Alinia (nitazoxanide). It was not one of the drugs in promising clinical trials that go back to the 1980s, but it does work against *M. avium* (the unknown cause).

In the mid-1990s clarithromycin alone was found able to put about 50 percent of patients in remission. Clarithromycin is a very powerful *macrolide* antibiotic, and I have a lot of respect for it. But it is difficult for some to take because after being on it for about three days, some people will develop an almost intolerable metallic taste in their mouth. I took it for dysentery once and could feel it working within minutes. A drug called azithromycin is less potent but also less prone to have an untoward side effect and may be a better option. A good clinical response to this drug is often the only clue that *M. avium* is the culprit.

The combination of the drugs that can be used in treatment has a few variations, but rifabutin (450 mg/d), clarithromycin (750 mg/d), and clofazimine (2 mg/kg/d) have been considered the core. Again, I would substitute azithromycin for clarithromycin, and ethambutol for clofazimine, because one of the side effects of clofazimine is skin discoloration, although the discoloration is not supposed to be permanent. We are talking about remission rates as high as 89 percent, and today I would add in Alinia (nitazoxinide) and keep patients on this course for a year.

Why don't gastroenterologists use this protocol, or something akin to it, despite the overwhelming evidence in the medical literature? Is there some austere body of sages who need to come forward and say, once and for all, that *M. avium* subspecies *paratuberculosis* is the cause of Crohn's disease?

Do your own verification. The conventional "wisdom" is that the causes of these diseases are unknown and the treatment consists of 1) aminosalicylate antibiotics (5-ASA and 4-ASA), because they are believed to be anti-inflammatory just like Dr. Kagan said; 2) corticosteroids, which will suppress the immune system; 3) immunomodulators that further suppress the immune system, such as Yervoy (ipilimumab); and 4) biological agents such as Enbrel (etanercept) or Humira (adalimumab).

Not much has changed since I went on rounds with Dr. Kagan over three decades ago except for the addition of biologics and immunomodulators, but neither treats the underlying infection, and if anything, they make the underlying infection worse. Both 4-ASA and 5-ASA will treat the infection as they are known to treat mycobacterium.

So, what is the holdup? As always, follow the money. Pharmaceutical companies can't make money treating anything with generic, off-patent drugs, but they can make money selling very expensive immunomodulators/biologics. And while they are making money selling something very expensive—even if that is the wrong thing to sell because it does not serve the patient—they will keep what they know about the disease to themselves unless you listen to the fine print.

Do you listen to fine print? Especially on those TV commercials selling drugs like Enbrel (etanercept) or Humira (adalimumab)? The fine print starts off by saying "patients treated with Enbrel are at increased risk for developing serious infections that may lead to hospitalization or death."

If you continue to listen, you will hear something like "if you have a serious infection like tuberculosis, this drug is not for you." Like tuberculosis . . . such as paratuberculosis? In other words, "If you have an infection, any infection, don't take Humira."

"Get tested for tuberculosis," they say.

Dollars to donuts, "they" know what causes Crohn's and the other IBDs—they just don't want you to know, and at the same time they want to wash their hands. It must allow them to sleep better at night. Again, the public should know that pharmaceutical corporations are not required to operate in the consumer's interest.

Physicians, patient support groups, and the general public seem to be totally unaware that pharmaceutical companies have a special interest in pretending that there is no known cause for many of the disorders we suffer from. They also have a special interest in helping the public ignore non-patentable therapies or off-patent therapies. The day will come when everyone has to admit, in the case of IBD, that it is mostly caused by an infection with *M. avium*. Just don't hold your sphincter waiting to hear any apologies.

Without fanfare, a new version of an old drug started being advertised on TV in 2015. Salix Pharmaceuticals holds a US patent for rifaximin and started marketing the drug under the name Xifaxan for IBS-D. Rifaximin is an antibiotic based on rifamycin, a drug used to treat mycobacterium—the same mycobacterium that is the "M" in MAP. They couldn't actually shout that out, because that might upset the apple cart and make others look stupid. Not good for business, especially when they want the very physicians who have been prescribing immunosuppressants to now prescribe their antibiotic. They have to be a little mysterious and indirect with the medical community who is deep into not knowing what causes IBS-D (CD and UC); although, they are willing to entertain that IBS-D patients may have bacterial overgrowth issues—just don't tell them MAP is the cause.

Don't you think it is weird how one pharmaceutical company will say they have an antibiotic to treat IBS-D, and another pharmaceutical company wants CD patients to take their immunospressive drug but warns you not to take it if you have a serious infection, like tuberculosis (a mycobacterium)? If anyone knows that MAP is the cause of IBS-D, it is a pharmaceutical company, because it is their business to know—unethical, isn't it?

I am aware of no evidence that rifaximin is any more effective than the off-patent rifamycins, such as rifabutin.

## GUT DYSBIOSIS, FLUORIDE, AND THE BLOOD-BRAIN BARRIER

I would like to believe that what happens in the gut (intestines) stays in the gut, but that is not true anymore than what happens in Las Vegas stays in Las Vegas. Glyphosate (see chapter 2), to name just one pesticide, causes a change in the types of bacteria that populate the human intestines and will lead to an overgrowth of *Clostridium difficile*, with its toxic by-product p-cresol, which enhances uptake of aluminum. Glyphosate itself allows Al to bypass the gut barrier, thereby increasing Al neurotoxicity.

Glyphosate is a serious endocrine disruptor that will cause deleterious changes to the uteruses of rats at doses considered safe in the United States.[164] One also wonders about all the food allergies we are now seeing, for if glyphosate substitutes itself for another amino acid, such as glycine, then you have a misfolded and messed up protein that the human body is not capable of digesting. This large protein then gets into the bloodstream and the immune system attacks it, so where there was once no allergy to soy, or corn, or wheat . . . now there is.

It is safe to say that the tangled web of synergetic toxicity from heavy metals and pesticides is so underappreciated, so misunderstood, and so completely dangerous that it threatens human life on this planet, as has been repeated so many times in this book. I apologize for constantly bringing up the 900-pound gorilla in the room, but he is really starting to smell.

There is a saying that just because you can do something doesn't mean you should do something. Just because you can build a nuclear reactor on an earthquake fault doesn't mean you should. In fact, if you do not know how to dispose of the dangerous waste you create, maybe you shouldn't be using that technology at all. But that is where the greed factor takes over and overrides what little sanity technocrats have.

In the case of fluoride, the powers that be came up with a great solution for disposing of a toxic industrial by-product—they turned it into a supplement that they claimed was not only good for our teeth, it was so good they would mandate that we drink it whether we wanted to or not—literally, this is mass medication of the masses, but why?

The German High Command in WWII intentionally fluoridated drinking water in certain areas to control the population. Even in extremely diluted amounts they knew that fluoride would affect the demeanor of those drinking it, making them docile and controllable. I can assure you they cared nothing about teeth except for the gold they wanted to extract from them.

Quoting Einstein's nephew, Dr. E. H. Bronner, a chemist who had also been a prisoner of war during WWII, in a letter printed in the *Catholic Mirror*, Springfield, Massachusetts, January 1952, he says:

It appears that the citizens of Massachusetts are among the "next" on the agenda of the water poisoners. There is a sinister network of subversive agents, Godless "intellectual" parasites, working in our country today whose ramifications grow more extensive, more successful and more alarming each new year and whose true objective is to demoralize, paralyze and destroy our great Republic—from within if they can, according to their plan—for their own possession.

The tragic success they have already attained in their long siege to destroy the moral fiber of American life is now one of their most potent footholds towards their own ultimate victory over us.

Fluoridation of our community water systems can well become their most subtle weapon for our sure physical and mental deterioration.

In the last twenty-two years as a research chemist of established standing, I built three American chemical plants and licensed six of my fifty-three patents. Based on my years of practical experience in the health-food and chemical field, let me warn you: fluoridation of drinking water is criminal insanity, sure national suicide. Don't do it.

Even in small quantities, sodium fluoride is a deadly poison to which no effective antidote has been found. Every exterminator knows that it is the most efficient rat-killer. Sodium fluoride is entirely different from organic calcium-fluoro-phosphate needed by our bodies and provided by nature, in God's great providence and love, to build and strengthen our bones and our teeth. This organic calcium-fluoro-phosphate, derived from proper foods, is an edible organic salt, insoluble in water and assimilable by the human body, whereas the non-organic sodium fluoride used in fluoridating water is instant poison to the body and fully water soluble. The body refuses to assimilate it.

Careful, bona fide laboratory experimentation by conscientious, patriotic research chemists, and actual medical experience, have both revealed that instead of preserving or promoting "dental health," drinking fluoridated water destroys teeth before adulthood and after by destructive mottling and other pathological conditions and creates many other very grave pathological conditions in the internal organisms. How can it be called a "health" plan?

That any so-called "doctors" would persuade a civilized nation to add voluntarily a deadly poison to its drinking water systems is unbelievable. It is the height of criminal insanity. No wonder Hitler and Stalin fully believed and agreed from 1939 to 1941 that, quoting from both Lenin's last will and Hitler's *Mein Kampf*: "America we shall demoralize, divide, and destroy from within."

Are our civil defense organizations and agencies awake to the perils of water poisoning by fluoridation? Its use has been recorded in other countries. Sodium fluoride water solutions are the cheapest and most effective rat killers known to chemists: colorless, odorless, tasteless; no antidote, no remedy, no hope; instant and complete extermination of rats.

Fluoridation of water systems can be slow national suicide, or quick national liquidation.

I know that most of the Americans reading this have recently brushed their teeth with fluoridated toothpaste. But why?

Fluoride is more toxic than lead. If some kid decided to sell homemade tooth-paste naturally sweetened with the good taste of lead, he would probably be arrested for poisoning people, but it is legal to put something even more toxic than lead in a product and tell consumers it is good for their teeth.

If a twenty-pound child were to eat the contents of a tube of toothpaste, do you know what the result would be? Death by fluoride!

First and foremost, show us the science, show us the independent research that shows drinking fluoride, or brushing one's teeth with fluoride, is good for one's body and teeth. Where is this science?

The claims are that drinking fluoridated water will reduce cavities 65 percent. These are just claims that were fed to us like slop, and we ate it. This is why "they" think we are so stupid. We don't question authority and when we don't, they stick it to us.

The truth is that modern studies have shown drinking fluoride reduces cavities by 0 percent:

> Lack of a significant relationship between consumption of nonpublic wa-ter and caries experience in the permanent dentition across any of the differing conditions of access to fluoridated tap water. [165]
>
> Results of recent large-scale studies in at least three countries show that, when similar communities are compared and the traditional DMFT index of dental caries is used, there is no detectable difference in caries prevalence. This has been demonstrated for schoolchildren in the major cities of New Zealand, Australia, the US and elsewhere.[166]

Why do we just blindly accept being experimented on and in many cases poisoned because some authority figure or agency says it is a good idea?

Why don't we demand solid, independent science in these public health mat-ters? Why do we accept the orders, laws, and commands from those we know are intellectually, ethically, and financially compromised by factions that can't be trusted?

Are we mice, or is there just something about not being able to challenge the fools that tell us what our reality should be?

We elect legislators who are practically bought and paid for by corporations, and we think we have a representative democracy. We don't have representation. We have puppets and lobbyists, and a media that is under their control. We have Corporatetocracy and Idiocracy. To quote D. H. Lawrence, "*Money is our madness, our vast collective madness.*"

# 5

# Traumatic Brain Injury, Multiple Sclerosis, and Hyperbaric Oxygen Therapy

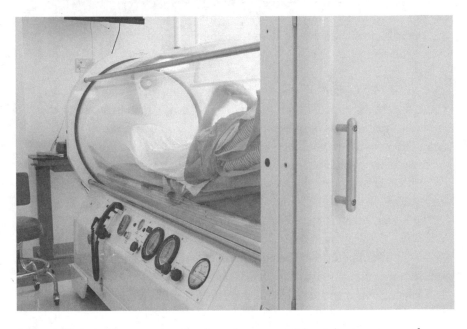

"Compelling evidence suggests the advantage of hyperbaric oxygen therapy (HBOT) in traumatic brain injury. . . . Patients undergoing hyperbaric therapy achieved significant improvement. . . . with a lower overall mortality, suggesting its utility as a standard intensive care regimen in traumatic brain injury."[167]

Hyperbaric oxygen therapy (HBOT) saturates the body's tissues with oxygen using a pressure vessel. HBOT is most often recognized as the treatment for decompression sickness (DCS) or "the bends." DCS causes significant neurological injury and post initial injury. The dysfunctional changes are virtually identical to those caused by trauma. Thus oxygen under pressure has been used to treat neurological injuries since 1937, almost eighty years. No one has found a replacement or substitute treatment for the bends that works as well as oxygen. HBOT results in a 95 percent acute treatment cure rate for DCS in all of the navies of the world. Combining HBOT with other therapies that help brain-injured patients enhances the effect of those treatments and makes these other therapies less costly, while creating additional recovery in any given patient.

An increase of one-half atmosphere will raise the oxygen levels in plasma seven times to twelve times normal (700 percent to 1,200 percent). Under this increased pressure, oxygen acts like a drug- and DNA-signaling agent. This treatment's mechanisms of action simply follow the general gas laws for saturating liquids with a gas, similar to the way SodaStream saturates water with carbon dioxide. No one yet has found a substitute for oxygen in human physiological processes, and any injury caused by a lack of oxygen can be expected to benefit from HBOT with the right oxygen dosage. Saturating with oxygen is a safe procedure when all of the correct protocols are followed, and significant side effects are extremely rare.

The history of hyperbaric medicine reaches back to the year 1620 when Drebbel developed a one-atmosphere diving bell, and forty years later Boyle joined forces with Gay-Lussac to develop the general gas law. Moving the sands of time to the near past, the modern age of hyperbaric medicine began in 1937 when Behnke and Shaw used a hyperbaric chamber to treat DCS. However, it was not until 1955 that there was major interest in using hyperbaric oxygenation (HBO) outside of treating DCS. That year, Churchill-Davidson began to use oxygen therapy in a hyperbaric chamber to treat the damage induced by radiotherapy in cancer patients.

In 1956, Boerema (Holland) performed the first reported heart surgery on "blue babies" in a hyperbaric chamber. He became the "Father of Hyperbaric Medicine" when he treated a woman who had been badly beaten, was unconscious, and was about to lose her leg. This became the first recorded prevention of an amputation with HBOT, and the woman did well. The next year his famous "Life without Blood" study was published. He referred to the treatment as "oxygen drenching."[168]

In 1962, Sharp and Smith (Scotland) were first to use HBOT to treat carbon monoxide poisoning; in 1963, Hitchcock testified before the House Labor Health, Education and Welfare Committee on the need for hyperbaric chambers in surgery, and Congress appropriated money for building a score of them.[169] In 1965, Perrins (United Kingdom) showed the effectiveness of HBOT in osteomyelitis, and in 1965, Japanese researchers treated the first burn patients.

In 1966, Saltzman et al. (United States) showed the effectiveness of HBOT in stroke patients; in 1970, Boschetty and Cernoch (Czechoslovakia) used HBOT to treat multiple sclerosis (MS). In 1971 Lamm (France) used HBOT for treatment of sudden deafness, and in 1973, Thurston showed that HBOT reduces mortality in myocardial infarction.

In 1976, Hollbach and Wasserman determined that 1.5 ATA (atmospheres absolute) maximizes oxygen content and glucose metabolism in the brain; in 1983, the first double-blind randomized control trial (RCT) was conducted using HBOT to treat MS. In 1987, Jain (Swiss) treated paralysis of stroke with HBOT. In 1989, the US Navy discovered that bubbles (nitrogen gas) are gone within five minutes, so while DCS is caused by bubbles initially, the secondary injury cascade is the same as in all brain insults.

In 1992, Harch treated the first delayed decompression sickness, which led to the treating of "dementia pugilistica" in boxers, children with cerebral palsy or autism, and nearly 700 patients with fifty various neurological conditions. Also in 1992, Rockswold (United States) conducted the first double-blind RCT showing that HBOT reduces mortality in acute traumatic brain injury (TBI) by 59 percent, the largest single reduction in mortality since the invention of the ambulance, the use of helicopters in Vietnam for battle casualties, and the use of penicillin for infection.

In 2002, a US Army study confirmed Harch's finding that HBOT repairs white matter damage in children with cerebral palsy (CP), and a Canadian group showed hyperbaric air (at 1.3 atmospheres), the original treatment for DCS and mountain sickness, and HBOT (at 1.75 atmospheres) effective in treating CP in double-blind randomized trial.

In 2005, I treated for the first time a child with fetal alcohol syndrome,[170] and Thom (United States) found that HBO causes stem cell mobilization. In 2007, Harch et al. (United States) treated chronic TBI in animal models, and in 2009 in military veterans;[171] in 2010, Godman discovered that HBOT activates 8,101 genes, reducing inflammation and increasing growth and repair hormones. In 2011, I treated the first retired National Football League (NFL) player treated for chronic traumatic encephalopathy (CTE);[172] in 2012, Harch demonstrated use of HBOT to treat blast-induced, post-concussion syndrome and post-traumatic stress disorder.

The above is not meant to be a comprehensive timeline, a meta-analysis of HBOT for various conditions, but rather an opportunity to understand why a benign yet beneficial therapy has been ignored and even treated with great disdain. Bureaucratic concerns have repeatedly trumped medical and scientific evidence. For someone with training in decision theory and bureaucratic behavior, the problems are very clear.

Each time in history when a decision was made about the deployment of hyperbaric oxygen therapy (starting with Behnke's discovery of oxygen improving the outcomes for DCS), bureaucratic concerns over budget constraints trumped science, to the determent of the persons those bureaucracies were intended to serve. Sometimes it was concerns about costs. Other times it was incorrect assumptions about the impact of the new science on the healthcare system. The latest concern is that the military fears that if HBOT was acknowledged as an official treatment for TBI/PTSD, then hordes of troops that were handling their injuries, because there was no viable alternative but to grin and bear it, would come out of the closet and reveal that they too had TBI/PTSD and in so doing decimate the military as a fighting force. Then again, maybe the Department of Defense (DoD) just wants to be able to justify mind-control cybernetic solutions to TBI/PTSD, and if HBOT were recognized as an efficacious therapy for this problem, then their cover is blown for doing who knows what to the brains of wounded soldiers in the name of mind-control.

There is no evidence of a pharmaceutical company running interference, although such interference could be inferred after a 1983 study was published in the *New England Journal of Medicine* showing HBOT to benefit patients with multiple sclerosis. B. H. Fischer, MD, a tenured professor at New York University, became the principal investigator of a study funded by the National Multiple Sclerosis Society (which is directly funded by pharmaceutical companies). Apparently, this society had great difficulty accepting the results of the work Dr. Fischer had completed, and multiple revisions were made to weaken the conclusions sufficiently to satisfy the editors of the *New England Journal of Medicine*. In this double-blind controlled study of patients with advanced chronic disabilities, Fischer found significant improvement in objective measurements, and the treatment effect persisted for at least one year.[173]

(Today, HBOT is the primary treatment in the United Kingdom for MS patients by MS patients—the National Health Service is not part of the program in treating MS patients with HBOT, nor do those who run the program want them to be.)

The study was never followed up, despite the positive results, for all the usual reasons. Clinical trials are expensive, and no one wants to fund a study with no monetary profit potential. So the treatment languished for lack of financial support and sponsorship. Indeed, Fischer lost his position, and his chamber was destroyed. (At the end of this chapter I will address MS.)

The reports about HBOT's impact on patients have never changed. What has changed is our understanding of the mechanisms of action and how vital oxygen is to healthy functioning human metabolism.

For example, a 2002 Canadian double-blind, randomized study[174] found that even room air under relatively low pressure (1.3 atmospheres) improved the clinical outcomes of children. Ten times more progress was made in gross motor function (GMF) during the two months of hyperbaric therapy (while all other therapies were ceased) than during the three months of follow-up with OT/PT restarted. The editorial in the *Lancet*, where the article was published, pointed out that "both groups of children improved substantially with respect to GMF, speech, attention, memory and functional skills." The Canadian government, which financed the study after being pressured by parents of children with cerebral palsy, falsely claimed the pressurized room air was a placebo and therefore there was no difference between the placebo group and the group of children receiving 100 percent oxygen. While this is sadly amusing, it kept HBOT from becoming standard of care for children with CP in Canada and in the United States. This is a gross tragedy and disservice, and not using hyperbaric oxygen therapy to treat these children when their brains are plastic and recovery can be dramatic leaves them as adults with continued high care costs and lost productivity.

HBOT has truly been the Cinderella of conventional medicine, which means it has been an attractive therapy that has shown itself to be efficacious in treating many conditions and yet is treated with derision or ignored at best. Because no patent is possible on oxygen (or any other element), there is no profit to spark a large pharmaceutical company's interest to prove or promote it. Few know about HBOT's effects on the body and medical conditions outside of diving medicine and wound care centers. But this has become much more than an issue of lack of marketing and poor public relations. With twenty US military veterans committing suicide every day directly related to TBI/PTSD, the lack of access to HBOT pushes this into the realm of criminality.

Suicide losses exceed combat casualties, and even National Football League (NFL) veterans are committing suicide. The clinical trial called the National Brain Injury Rescue and Rehabilitation project[175] showed HBOT can virtually eliminate suicidality in this population once they are treated with HBOT, while reducing depression by 51 percent. That is a larger and broader effect on depression than anything advertised on television. Yet even on the basis of compassionate use, it is not possible to get HBOT paid for to treat TBI even though HBOT has more "on-label" indications for brain injury than any other drug or therapy in medicine. The issue at hand is not whether HBOT is effective for treating TBI/PTSD; that has been proven. The issue is the interference. People are dying because they are not getting into hyperbaric chambers to breathe oxygen. The time is upon us to expose the obfuscation of this humanitarian therapy.

In 2009, and again in 2010, Paul Harch, MD, Director of the LSU Hyperbaric Medicine Department, delivered testimony to both the House and Senate Armed Services Committees reminding them that the epidemic of suicides among military veterans was most likely due to cocktail of "off-label" antidepressants they were being prescribed—black-boxed antidepressants, none of which are approved for treating TBI. Others have delivered this warning as well. The exact FDA warning states: "Antidepressants increased the risk compared to placebo of suicidal thinking and behavior (suicidality) in children, adolescents, and young adults in short-term studies of major depressive disorder (MDD) and other psychiatric disorders. Anyone considering the use of [insert name of antidepressant] or any other antidepressant in a child, adolescent, or young adult must balance this risk with the clinical need."[176]

While antidepressants are modestly effective in reducing the symptoms of severe depression, they increase the brain's susceptibility to future episodes after they have been discontinued. This fact contradicts pharmaceutical company–sponsored research. Antidepressants cause neuronal damage and cause mature neurons to revert to an immature state, both of which may explain why antidepressants also cause neurons to undergo apoptosis (programmed death).[177] If antidepressants cause death on a micro level, then it is much easier to understand why certain patients commit suicide given that the human body (macro level) is made up of these cells. Not only are black-boxed, off-label selective serotonin reuptake inhibitors (SSRIs) prescribed to a vulnerable population, but they are done so without any regard to an ability to metabolize this class of drugs,[178] which further exacerbates suicidal behaviors. And then it seems SSRIs actually deplete both catecholamine and serotonin,[179] which is exactly what isn't in a depressed individual's interest. Serotonin makes humans feel happy and relaxed, and catecholamines, such as the neurotransmitter dopamine, help one feel less agitated.

Up against black-boxed antidepressants that are not efficacious, it should be a no-brainer to treat those who have received a TBI with a safe, off-label drug—that is, oxygen at hyperbaric doses—after two decades of use treating various neurological conditions. So what is the problem? What does it take to become "standard-of-care"?

As already pointed out, HBOT is non-patentable. Research on non-patentable or off-patent drugs or with those with insufficient marketing prospects (orphan drugs) is funded by nonprofit or charitable organizations only. Drugs for which a patent cannot be granted are not being developed or marketed, even when they respond to a public health need. Patients, physicians, and other caregivers consequently cannot take advantage of potentially effective treatments—they can't even find out about them.

But while HBOT won't make any entity large profits, doesn't it have other monetary incentives? For each active-duty brain-injured solider returned to duty, the lifetime savings to the government is $2.6 million and $2 million for each injured service member returned to work or school. Between 60 percent and 80 percent of the veterans participating in the National Brain Injury Rescue and Rehabilitation (NBIRR) project returned to work, duty, or school after receiving HBOT. One would think that would move the powers that be to action, but it has not. And the reason for that has already been pointed out: the DoD doesn't want to acknowledge there is a safe and efficacious therapy for TBI/PTSD because they fear so many troops would want to receive this therapy as to decimate an impractical number of troops. The NFL provides an example of this on a smaller scale.

For many decades, evidence has linked repetitive traumatic brain injury to long-term neurological problems in many sports. The NFL, as the organizer, marketer, and face of the most popular sport in the United States, in which head trauma is a regular occurrence, was aware of the evidence and the risks associated with repetitive traumatic brain injuries and concussions for decades, but it apparently ignored, and worse, actively concealed, the information from those who participated in organized football at all levels.

Apparently the NFL inserted itself into the scientific research and discussion concerning the relationship between concussions and short-term and long-term impairment of the brain. After doing so, the NFL then intentionally and fraudulently misled present and former players, and all people who reasonably relied upon the NFL's expertise about its own sport regarding the short-term and long-term risks posed by concussions and head trauma.

Rather than warn players that they risked permanent brain injury if they returned to play too soon after sustaining a concussion, the NFL actively deceived players by misrepresenting to them that concussions did not present serious, life-altering risks. Plaintiffs in the various brain injury law cases have accused the NFL of withholding knowledge allegedly in their possession related to the possibility of brain injury and concealing such concerns. "Rather than warn players that they risked permanent brain injury if they returned to play too soon after sustaining a concussion, the NFL actively deceived players, by misrepresenting to them that concussions did not present serious, life-altering risks." [180]

The NFL created the Mild Traumatic Brain Injury Committee (the MTBI Committee) in 1994 to research and ameliorate the impact of concussions on NFL players. Notwithstanding the purported purpose of the MTBI Committee, and despite clear medical evidence that on-field concussions led directly to brain injuries with tragic results for players at every level of the sport, the NFL failed to inform its current and former players of the true risks associated with such head trauma and purposefully misrepresented and/or concealed medical evidence on that issue. The NFL also stonewalled on an intervention and therapy that could have helped injured players, regardless of whether those injuries were acute or chronic. The author has firsthand experience dealing with the NFL's 88 Plan in an attempt to get veteran NFL players with dementia HBOT.

The 88 Plan is designed to assist players who are vested under the Bert Bell/Pete Rozelle NFL Player Retirement Plan and who are diagnosed as having dementia. But if a plan member tries to get HBOT using the plan because they have been diagnosed with CTE, they will be told CTE does not cause dementia, and therefore HBOT, which treats CTE, will not be a covered benefit. Obviously, that is irrational, but there is often madness behind the reason for not allowing an effective treatment to be utilized by those who need it. In the case of military veterans, avoiding twenty suicides every day might be seen as a tremendous cost savings to certain decision makers. Be that as it may, the DoD can't have an unknown throng of troops suddenly declare they have TBI/PTSD too should HBOT be embraced.

This is truly misanthropic, but no moreso than what tobacco corporations do, and we still tolerate their malfeasance. In the case of the NFL, the reason for prevaricating about TBI and potential treatments is just a business decision. The exposure of the "hit squad" of the New Orleans Saints, where there was a bounty put on players from opposing teams (to cause injury on the field), is a clear example of what kind of business this is about.

A great deal of time has been lost by those who believe hyperbaric oxygen either is a placebo or should be subjected to placebo-controlled studies, or want others to believe so. But oxygen can never be a placebo. HBOT is an FDA-approved drug that affects nonspecific biological repair; in fact, it is the only nonhormonal FDA-approved treatment known to repair and regenerate human tissue. It does so at a DNA level by activating growth factors and reviving mitochondrial function.[181] The beneficial effects of HBOT apply no matter where a wound or injury is located in the body.

The DoD-funded HBOT studies used pressurized air as their placebos, knowing that pressurized air is not a placebo and has been shown to be therapeutic. Their hopeful delusion was that since so few know anything about HBOT, they could get away with this piece of fraud. So, all DoD-funded studies seem to come out with negative results, whereas all civilian studies come out with positive results.

In the last decade, many peer-reviewed articles have been published that demonstrate HBOT is effective at repairing an injured brain even long after that injury took place. One of the most notable used only one-half of the NBIRR protocol (forty 60-minute treatments at 1.5 atmospheres). The blast-induced TBI war veterans experienced a 15-point IQ increase ($p < 0.001$), a 39 percent reduction in post-concussion symptoms, a 30 percent reduction in PTSD symptoms, and a 51 percent decrease in depression. This is all consistent with past-published reports of HBOT in chronic brain injury, including research by the US Army on brain-injured children.[182]

The first battle casualty to be treated with HBOT (at 1.5 atmospheres), and one of the few to be treated, was General Patt Maney (retired) for his blast-induced brain injury in Afghanistan. His treatment was ordered after nine months of therapy at Walter Reed had shown minimal improvement. As a result of his injuries, he was nonfunctional and unable to return to his job, let alone redeploy to Afghanistan. After HBOT treatment he was discharged from Walter Reed and returned to his civilian job as a Florida state judge.

He received treatment from George Washington University Medical Center at the Tricare Reimbursement rate of $250 per treatment. Counting lost time and hospital costs, and his months at Walter Reed making no progress, the DoD spent $400,950, with a permanent disability loss to the service of $1.3 million. Had he received HBOT earlier, he would have been able to remain on active duty, a savings of $1.3 million, but more importantly, the five months of recovery once he began receiving HBOT cost $133,650, a savings to the government of $287,300. No other patients were treated at the Walter Reed's brain injury center, despite the general's remarkable recovery that everyone on the staff witnessed. The $20,000 for his hyperbaric medical treatment was $12,000 less than what a RAND report states the annual ongoing costs per year of the current treatments for mild-TBI is,[183] and that is a lot of SSRIs.

Since every working person represents $1 million in tax revenue over their working life to the government, that government should be interested in and foster payment for biological repair of brain injury. Thus every brain-injured veteran, all 700,000+ of them, at a cost of $60,000 per year to the economy every year in increased costs and lost productivity, is a $42 billion drain on the economy. Treated, they immediately set about doing what young people do: they begin to form families and create the next American generation. Injured, they are unable to do so. It is highly likely that these untreated brain injuries are a major cause of our nation's economic challenges. But bureaucracies' ability to think laterally is limited. When Medicare approved HBOT to treat diabetic foot ulcers at the end of 2002, they made it available only for Wagner III and IV lesions (osteomyelitis and gangrene), so afraid were they of budgetary constraints.

HBOT prevents 75 percent of major limb amputations in Wagner III and IV ulcers, but if they had included Wagner II lesions, HBOT would be preventing 88 percent of amputations. There are a lot of unnecessary amputations, not because of bad science, but because technocrats were afraid of having a short-term budget problem.

HBOT is an efficacious, benign, and humanitarian way to affect brain repair, but it has not been adopted because it lacks patent protection and has no large corporate sponsors. It has also met interference because other agendas are present, be they the protection of the status quo, myopic budgetary constraints, or perceived liability issues. After all, when you treat TBI directly the way that HBOT does, the problems creating those TBIs in the first place are harder to ignore, and the unconscious way those problems have been dealt with are harder to deny. It brings the true cost and repercussions of war to the fore, and football, after all, is just a form of organized war.

This perspective, should it be adopted by the general public, will be a catalyst for change. So, whether that means changing the way football is played to not allowing our "leaders" to guide us into unending military forays for the sake of war-profiting run amok—all of these subterrain issues come into play when a very straightforward and effective therapy tries to assert itself: hence the resistance both on a conscious and a subconscious level.

Veterans are considered a threat by the security apparatus in the United States. They are considered a threat because many know what is really going on; that is, our troops are being used to feed conflict so others can profit. Is someone thinking that it is better to let twenty potential threats kill themselves every day? This is a dark rabbit hole to go down, but the human cost of war is a deep rabbit hole and one that many want to keep hidden. Someone is making money when someone else bleeds to death from a cluster bomb. It is that black and white—someone is making money giving dangerous SSRIs to treat TBI.

Technocrats rotating between corporation and state are the last people you want making medical decisions, but that is exactly who has been making medical decisions. These are all things to be looked at when asking the question, why is a therapy like HBOT being suppressed? If the man on the street understood why certain medical therapies are not available while other dangerous and non-efficacious therapies are favored, then change would be demanded.

Right now the man on the street is being kept in the dark about how money drives medical decisions to the extent it is today and about what lengths will be taken should something come forward that could interfere with the flow of that money.

## MORE ON MULTIPLE SCLEROSIS

Multiple sclerosis (MS) is a chronic inflammatory demyelinating disease of the central nervous system (CNS) causing progressive disability. Literally, the name just refers to the multiple scars seen in the brain on scans. (Lyme is often misdiagnosed as MS, but this section is about real MS.)

In many academic circles (as opposed to clinical circles where physicians treat patients), there is little doubt that the majority of MS victims have a viral infection, and the most commonly recognized association has been with the EBV variety.[184] There are other possible infectious agents implicated, because remember: it is never just one thing. But the EBV association is undeniable.[185] Just as Lyme can activate a latent EBV infection, maybe EBV really is only an association—a party guest, but not the virus that pulls the trigger. Maybe the real viral trigger is another virus!

In 2011, a study[186] was published looking at a population of almost 20,000 between the years 1998 and 2005. The study found that those living near areas of high pesticide use had an increased risk of neurodegenerative diseases—everything from AD and MS to psychiatric problems, including suicide attempts.

There is clear evidence that pesticide exposure at relatively low doses affects brain cells and causes cancer and ailments too numerous to list.

The European Commission on July 12, 2006, in relation to EU Thematic Strategy on pesticides, acknowledged, "Long term exposure to pesticides can lead to serious disturbances to the immune system, sexual disorders, cancers, sterility, birth defects, damage to the nervous system and genetic damage."

Warnings regarding the links between pesticides and chronic diseases can be found in many peer-reviewed scientific journals. But the government has done less than nothing in many cases by allowing things like dicofol to be used while claiming DDT has been banned. They—the CDC, FDA, EPA, USDA—can't be trusted. None of them.

The only answer is the widespread adoption of truly sustainable nonchemical and natural methods as an alternative to chemical pesticides. As consumers we can make this change. We can make this happen. It will be the only way, as "the system" is broken—completely and utterly broken.

What is stopping physicians from understanding that, for the most part, MS is likely viral encephalitis triggered by environmental factors (pesticides)?

The same thing keeping them from understanding that IBD is caused, for the most part, by *M. avium*. A corporation(s) is making a lot of money treating MS with expensive drugs that don't address the infectious disease issue.

If MS were a viral infection, then would HIV-positive patients be less likely to get MS given that HIV patients are almost always on antiviral drugs? Or if they had MS and started getting treated for their HIV, wouldn't their MS go away?

Indeed! That is exactly what happens.[187]

Retroviruses (viruses that use RNA as their genetic material instead of DNA; HIV is a retrovirus) have been linked with MS.

In 2013, records of a cohort of Danish people with HIV compared to HIV-negative people were examined.[188] The study found a lower incidence of MS in people with HIV, but the incidence was not large enough to reach a statistically significant conclusion.

But another study, also done in 2013[189] in the UK, looked at the longitudinal hospital records of over 21,000 HIV-positive patients and nearly 5.3 million age- and sex-matched HIV-negative individuals between the years 1999 and 2011. The records were examined for a subsequent diagnosis of MS that might have occurred after the first mention of HIV in the record.

The records showed that the HIV-positive individuals showed a statistically significant lower incidence of MS in comparison to the HIV-negative individuals. In the HIV group, seven people developed MS, equating to a risk reduction of nearly two-thirds the expected rate.

It was assumed the vast majority were receiving combination antiretroviral therapy (cART). But without this treatment information, the authors were unable to conclude whether it is the treatment for HIV or the HIV infection itself that is protective against MS.

Which brings us to HGRV (human gamma retrovirus)—an endogenous/exogenous retrovirus (ERV). A controversial class of virus to be sure, but its existence is not controversial, yet there is hubris surrounding the potential danger of any virus that might find itself being a contaminant in a vaccine. Since "vaccines are safe and save lives," or so we are repeatedly told, then any virus found in a vaccine is either benign or of no concern to humans. It is like magic: if you are a virus, benign or not, but you want to be classified as being benign(ish), just get yourself found as a contaminant in vaccines.

The following was posted on an FDA website,[190] updated in February 2015: "A derivative of a mouse gammaretrovirus was used for gene therapy given to children in two clinical trials in Europe for X-linked severe combined immunodeficiency disease (X-SCID, more commonly known as the 'Bubble Boy Disease'). Although this therapy appeared to provide clinical benefit to most of the children, some patients developed the blood cancer leukemia. This demonstrated that these animal viruses can cause disease in humans, although except for the X-SCID clinical trials, gammaretroviruses used for gene therapy have not caused cancer."

That is so reassuring: except for the X-SCID trial, gammaretroviruses have not been found to cause cancer when used for gene therapy. I'll bet you those lucky buggers must have found their way into some vaccines to get such a stellar report. So glad they aren't causing cancer (yet), but what about other diseases, like MS?

After all, there is a hurt of problems between being 100 percent healthy and having cancer.

Lo and behold, ERVs are found in vaccines.[191] The retrovirus avian leukosis is found in the measles vaccine. A virus similar to simian retrovirus was identified in RotaTeq. Significant levels of porcine cirovirus 1 were found in Rotarix.

Now, it should go without saying that if vaccine manufacturers, who have no liability and total immunity, were to realize that viral contaminants are acceptable in their products (for whatever justification), then that leads to a very slippery slope where the shores of safety recede even further into the distance. Vaccine manufacturers realize this and are more than willing to exploit their lack of ability to produce a safe product.

Not all countries act like lemmings and follow the United States' lead in this arena. Japan has banned the MMR and taken Gardasil off the list of recommended vaccines. In China, if a few babies die from a vaccine, they will close down production, as they did when seventeen babies died from the Hep B vaccine. In the United States, the vaccine-injury reporting system has 1,000 babies reported dead as a result of the Hep B vaccine, but the response has been to try to take away parental rights for refusing vaccines. There seems to be more medical freedom in countries like Cuba and China than in the United States.

Never should we give up freedom of choice to an external authority. Informed consent should be the law of the land, but sadly it is not.

## TREATMENT OPTIONS

In the UK, HBOT is the primary treatment for MS by MS patients as previously pointed out. There are now over sixty charity centers treating MS patients and over 100 hyperbaric chambers throughout the UK doing this. It changes the clinical course of the illness, although it is not a cure. By improving immune-system function, HBOT helps the body's immune system fight off just about any infection without ever knowing what that infection might be. It is that simple.

If one were to add in omega-3s (the primary fat in the brain); B vitamins (especially biologically active $B_{12}$); curcumin (because it is neuroprotective); and the right mix of antiviral agents, I think an MS patient might be pleasantly surprised with the results.

Pairing Alinia along with a drug like ribavirin, which has been done when treating Hep C, and acyclovir, the active metabolite of valacyclovir (active against the herpes virus family), should be an adequate cocktail for most, especially if HBOT is being utilized at the same time. The first patient with MS I treated with ribavirin had Lyme, so first I treated her for her Lyme. When she still had MS symptoms after her Lyme treatment, I kept her on Alinia and added in the ribavirin (I already had her on valacyclovir, as her EBV titers were high). In her first week alone on ribavirin, her symptoms resolved by 50 percent. Adding in the ribavirin was key to changing the clinical course of her MS. Some clinicians use the HIV drugs Truvada and Isentress, but take note that results may not be overly dramatic at first because some MS patients are so vitally depleted they can't repair the damage right away even if the virus has been stopped.

In 2003, a research team conducted experiments using Dark Agouti rats.[192] Experimental autoimmune encephalomyelitis (EAE) induced in susceptible strains of rats is considered the best available model for studying events in MS, and their findings suggested that ribavirin attenuates experimental autoimmune encephalomyelitis (animal model of multiple sclerosis) by limiting cytokine-mediated immuno-inflammatory events that lead to central nervous system destruction.

When scientists don't realize they are dealing with an infection, finding an intervention that works is always attributed to having an effect on inflammation.

I bring up that rat study using ribavirin as back up for what I did clinically in a human, and while I am not saying ribavirin doesn't limit cytokine inflammation, I do think it is attacking the source of the inflammation as well—the retrovirus that no one seems to want to acknowledge as something that should be treated.

There is enough evidence that MS associated retrovirus is probably the cause of progressive MS, and this information has been around for well over a decade. In 2013, a review was published in BMC Neurology by Kari K. Nissen et al. entitled "Endogenous retroviruses and multiple sclerosis–new pieces to the puzzle."[193] These scientists consider MS an autoimmune disease, but the medical literature strongly suggests that the human endogenous retroviruses (HERVs) is "playing a role in the disease."

## MORE ON RHEUMATOID ARTHRITIS (RA)

Microorganisms, such as mycoplasmas, often lay dormant, waiting for conditions to be favorable for propagation. Remember, it is never just one thing, but what does the body do when it finds it can't kill an invader? In certain situations, it tries to wall it off, quarantine the organism using fibrin and the debris of inflammation to surround the mycoplasma for months to years—the disfiguring nodules of RA.

Mycoplasmas are capable of long-term survival inside our cells, waiting, perhaps, for some event that decreases our immune system's functionality, which also explains how symptoms come and go in waves.

Given that the medical community can't seem to wrap itself around the idea that RA is an infection, the usual treatment is anti-inflammatory drugs, but mycoplasma are facultative anaerobes, just like *Borrelia*. They are probably sensitive to changes in barometric pressure, triggering a migration to less-oxygenated areas, and this swarming triggers a cytokine or inflammatory response from the immune system. Hyperbaric oxygen treatments force oxygen into compromised cells and tissue, thus allowing the infection-fighting function of white blood cells to proceed.[194] HBOT is synergistic with antibiotics and acts as a direct antibiotic to anaerobic and facultative anaerobic bacteria. It should come as no surprise that there are studies in the medical literature supportive of using HBOT to treat RA: "In the patients with rheumatoid arthritis under HBO therapy the SOD activity was increased, whereas lipoperoxide values was decreased. Furthermore, ESR and Lansbury's index showed a remarkable recovery. These results suggest that HBO therapy may be an effective treatment for the patients with rheumatoid arthritis."[195]

"Regular" labs can't do comprehensive mycoplasma testing. There are labs, such as Clongen (www.clongen.com), that can test for multiple species. The reason to bring this up is that if a mycoplasma infection has hunkered down in one's body, it could mean a good six months of one or two antibiotics, such as doxycycline, and then rounds of six-week courses broken up by two-week breaks. It would be nice if some of these infections could be solved with a ten-day course of this or that, but the truth is, they can't.

# 6

# Mercury in Medicine: Quacks, Quackery, and Quacksalber

*"Penicillin sat on my shelf for twelve years while I was called a quack. I can only think of the thousands who died needlessly because my peers would not use my discovery."*

—Dr. Alexander Fleming

Mercury, the most toxic nonradioactive element on the periodic table, is called *Quecksilber* in German, which was the language of medicine for several hundred years. The bloodletting physicians of the Middle Ages used mercury extensively and, rightly so, they were called "quacks" (a fraudulent physician or a scam artist). I find the term is also inappropriately used against physicians who threaten the status quo where conventional medicine makes money from keeping things just the way they are (including the continued use of mercury in medicine). Since the conventional quacks are now the ones in charge, anyone who is against mercury in medicine has become the quack—it is part of the Orwellian doublespeak to which we are constantly being subjected.

In that letter I wrote to Senator Boxer I referred to the meeting I had with Jim Pirkle, PhD, at the CDC in 2006 (Dr. Pirkle helped get lead out of gasoline). I brought him the data I had collected on children whom I had tested for heavy metals. I showed Dr. Pirkle and his crew how a provocative urine toxic-metal test, where I gave them a chelating agent (DMSA), compared with the children's ability to perform on a standardized neurocognitive test. The higher the lead levels were in the urine, the poorer the performance. Then I showed them the improvement once I was able to get that lead out of their bodies.

The purpose of my meeting with him was to get the CDC seal of approval for doing the provocative urine toxic-metal test. Dr. Pirkle said he approved of it, but he said that to get the CDC seal of approval, they would have to do a study. They would go to New Mexico, do a study, and publish it. I met with the Secretary of the Environment at the time, and he said he was supportive but for one thing: he wanted a guarantee that if he invited the CDC to the state, whatever they ended up doing wouldn't cost the state of New Mexico any money. Well, I couldn't give him that guarantee—what if they found half the residents were full of lead or arsenic at levels that required medical attention, for example.

The study never happened, but at the end of that initial meeting I had at the CDC National Environmental Health Lab, several scientists rushed up to me and said that their real concern was mercury far more than lead. I had purposefully brought only cases of children who showed elevated lead without elevated mercury. I figured the CDC was no place to discuss the dangers of mercury, given they were so supportive of injecting it into all of the world's children. That was before I found out that it is only the Infectious Disease Division that is so enamored with giving the world's children mercury by injection (along with aluminum, etc.). But as Dr. Pirkle told me, the Infectious Disease Division made the policy and controlled the funding for all other divisions at the CDC.

Mercury poisoning is not at the root of all the world's evils, but it is among the top three. One in six women in the United States has mercury levels in the cord blood of their babies that is so high[196] that it will cause decreased IQ and neurological issues for their babies. Children with cord mercury $\geq 7.5$ µg/L are four times as likely to have an IQ score below 80, the clinical cutoff for borderline intellectual disability.[197]

When you understand that these poisons are synergistic with each other, so that a little of this and a little of that ends up being a whole lot of something that is much worse than the additive properties of any one poison, and you understand that these fools at the various federal agencies either don't understand or don't want to understand or are ordered not to understand, then you begin to appreciate why the projected frequency of autism in the United States by 2025 is expected to be one in two children.

If this were actually true, which it very well could turn out to be if current rates continue, then it should be upsetting to even the most apathetic among us, unless all the fluoridated water, aspartame, lead, aluminum, DDT, DDE, glyphosate, and mercury has finally done its job, and we are ripe for the culling of the global elite have had in store for us all along.

Aluminum (Al) has been mentioned several times, and when most people hear the word *aluminum* they think about cookware and aluminum foil, which are relatively benign products. But Al is not benign when you breathe it in or have it injected into the body.

Aluminum disrupts biological self-ordering, energy transduction, and signaling systems, thus increasing biosemiotic entropy.[198] Biosemiotics describes a process of understanding life in the context of the many different systems under which it operates. For example, if you have vaccine manufacturers put together a toxic concoction without any consideration of how these various toxic ingredients interact with each other or with the biological systems they are being injected into, then you have a lack of biosemiotics. Entropy in this context is about disorder, so Al increases a biological system's disorder.

Aluminum has been known as a toxicant for a hundred years: It injures both the brain and the immune systems, individually and synergistically. It disrupts DNA and RNA—the very coding of life. It destroys hydrogen bonds, literally ungluing living systems. It interferes with biological signaling—biosemiosis—from the very lowest to the highest levels in the nervous system, and last but not least its effects are synergistic with other toxicants, including mercury, lead, fluoride, and glyphosate.

It is easier to understand the tragedy of one than it is to understand the pathos of millions, so consider the story of the actor and dancer Buddy Ebsen, who was cast as the Tin Man in the 1939 production of the *Wizard of Oz*. He went through all the rehearsals and knew all the songs. But when they applied the Al dust makeup to him, it almost killed him. It is recorded as an allergic reaction, but it was not. It was Al toxicity from breathing in the dust. Don't go looking for Buddy in the movie because he isn't in it; he was too busy recovering from being poisoned.

Breathing in Al or being injected with Al is decidedly unhealthy and can be lethal. It makes you wonder why "they" are spraying from the skies aluminum, barium, strontium, and SF6 sulfur hexafloride.

If you keep eating, drinking, and breathing these elements, they will eventually be lethal. Call it chemtrails, Operation Indigo Skyfold, geoenginering, or whatever. One has to wonder whose idea this was, and what the heck did they think they were doing? Does it matter how well-intentioned geoengineering is if you have to do it with megatons of poison? The Tower of Babel was well intentioned, but look where that got us.

"Stratospheric aerosol injection (SAI), a method of seeding the stratosphere with particles that can help reflect the sun's heat, in much the same way that volcanic eruptions do."[199] That was a quote from CIA Director John O. Brennan to the Council on Foreign Relations, and was transcribed and uploaded to the CIA's official website on June 29, 2016. "Another example is the array of technologies—often referred to collectively as geoengineering—that potentially could help reverse the warming effects of global climate change. One that has gained my personal attention . . . An SAI program could limit global temperature increases, reducing some risks associated with higher temperatures and providing the world economy additional time to transition from fossil fuels. The process is also relatively inexpensive—the National Research Council estimates that a fully deployed SAI program would cost about $10 billion yearly."

You have to read between the lines because he does not come right out and say the CIA is involved in ongoing SAI pilot projects. After all, if you do something like this covertly, you can't be trusted, and the CIA is beyond reproach, so they certainly couldn't be involved.

SAI composition probably varies as various substances are tried out for various reasons, in various pilot projects and some probably have nothing to do with manipulating weather.

I can hear it all now: "We were doing this for the Greater Good, and how were we to know something untoward [fill in the blank] was going to happen?" Brennan went on to say, "On the technical side, greenhouse gas emission reductions would still have to accompany SAI to address other climate change effects, such as ocean acidification, because SAI alone would not remove greenhouse gases from the atmosphere." But decreasing the world's surplus population (the culling) will help decrease greenhouse gases, eh?

If you want to do your own due diligence, look at a website that lists all the Department of Energy's Climate Research Facility's (ARM's) ongoing aerosol projects.[200] In 2013, the UN's Intergovernmental Panel on Climate Change came right out and said the world wouldn't cool without geoengineering. Period.

Our government would never engage in a covert project on such a grand scale and keep it a secret like the "Manhattan Project." Although intentions have a way of being set in stone, so to speak, such as the Georgia Guidestones.[201] Some very wealthy, deluded people spent a pretty penny in 1980 to erect a monument that weighs a quarter of a million pounds of granite in Elbert County, Georgia. From what I understand, the culling needs to be focused in the good old United States because we are the ones who could stop this if we knew about it.

The very first commandment on the monument reads, "Maintain humanity under 500,000,000 in perpetual balance with nature." That means they want to reduce the current population of the planet by 73 percent, but there are only so many ways to do that. You can poison people, make them infertile, make them so sick they are not viable breeders, kill them in war or other form of violence, or unleash biological agents. It's hard to simply dismiss this when there are UN officials, such as Christiana Figueres, the Executive Secretary of the United Nations Framework Convention on Climate Change (UNFCC), openly talking about reducing the world's population.[202]

One just can't make this up. I am not saying that those behind these Guidestones are behind SAI. After all, the chemtrail project is on a very grand scale, but whatever they are doing, they are doing it in secret. And they clearly don't know

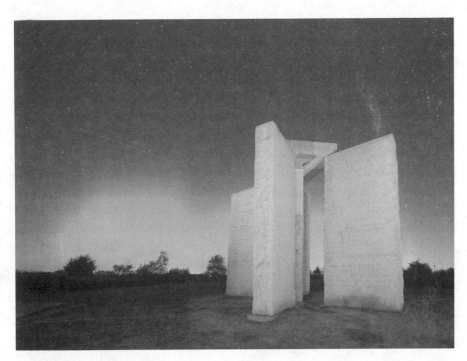

The Georgia Guidestones.

what they are doing, or they wouldn't be spraying parts of the Northern Hemisphere with who-knows-what. The Guidestones were blown apart by someone in 2022.

The SAI project affects every living thing on earth. It was never approved by any process that would allow for impact statements, etc. Can you imagine the public outcry if the public knew what was being sprayed and how toxic it is? Who gave them the right to do this?

Divide and conquer, mass shootings, riot in the streets, be they race riots or food riots, they just don't care—it is all about imposing control.

Keep watching football, staring at Kim Kardashian's butt, and having anxiety about how you are going to pay next month's rent. You won't have time to see what is taking place in the skies above or in the water below, which brings us to Minamata Bay.

## WELCOME TO MINAMATA BAY

As a young lad I would watch *The Wonderful World of Disney* on television. I loved listening to the Irish crooner on the Gulf Oil commercial, one of the show's major sponsors, sing, "Pulling into Bantry Bay bringing home d'oil." One day the commercials vanished. An oil tanker named *Betelgeuse* had caught fire and exploded while it was offloading in Bantry Bay.

These events are tragic, and the loss of life adds to the pathos, but strictly focusing on the oil itself, there are microorganisms in the sea that will eventually biodegrade the oil. The earth has periodically leaked oil here and there for eons of time, and opportunistic life adapted itself to work with that. Not making excuses for either oil spills or the exploitation of this resource without really understanding what it is—the earth's blood in a sense—but that is for a discussion on meta-earth science.

Deliberately pouring a nonbiodegradable material into waterways, looking the other way, and then lying about it is a whole other matter.

Over 3,000 victims have been recognized as having Minamata disease, the result of the Chisso Corporation dumping twenty-seven tons of mercury compounds into Minamata Bay, Japan, from 1932 to 1968. Thousands of people whose normal diet included fish from the bay unexpectedly developed symptoms of methylmercury poisoning. It is known that all forms of mercury are neurotoxic, especially during brain development.[203] By the mid-1950s, Minamata residents were diagnosed as having degeneration of their nervous systems. Numbness and other neuropathies occurred in their limbs and lips. Their speech became impeded and they experienced visual disturbances as well. Some lost consciousness while others developed extrapyramidal symptoms (involuntary movements). Meanwhile, cats were committing suicide and birds dropped dead on the wing. The Chisso Corporation denied all accusations that the mercury they were dumping was causing any illness, and they continued their pollution. By 1958, Chisso Corporation transferred their dumping from the Minamata Bay to the Minamata River in an inane attempt to mitigate the disaster they had created. The Minamata River flows past the town Hachimon and into the Shiranui Sea, and after a few months, the people of this area also began developing symptoms.

In July 1959, researchers from Kumamoto University concluded that organic mercury was the cause of Minamata disease. A number of committees, of which Chisso Corporation employees were members, formed to research the problem. The committees denied this information and refuted the direct link of mercury to the brain damage, gross deformities, and death caused to the citizens of Minamata and Niigata. Chisso deliberately concealed their own research implicating mercury as the cause of the disease, and it was only a deathbed confession by one of Chisso's own researchers that led to a 1973 verdict against the corporation.[204]

## AUTISM—A MERCURY ENCEPHALOPATHY?

Prior to receiving multiple (nine) vaccines in one office visit, Hannah Poling was a normally developing child. She did not have an existing encephalopathy. She was compensated by HHS for her resulting vaccine-induced medical problems including autism. She was found to have mitochondrial dysfunction after she regressed into autism—mitochondrial dysfunction is common among children on the autism spectrum. Julie Gerberding, present head of Merck's vaccine division, spoke to Sanjay Gupta on the Hannah Poling case when she was still head of the Centers for Disease Control: "Now, we all know that vaccines can occasionally cause fevers in kids. So if a child was immunized, got a fever, had other complications from the vaccines, and if you're predisposed with the mitochondrial disorder, it can certainly set off some damage. Some of the symptoms can be symptoms that have characteristics of autism."

At an event sponsored by the Groton Wellness organization in 2014, Stephanie Seneff of the Massachusetts Institute of Technology (MIT) said, "At today's rate, by 2025, one in two children will be autistic."

Autism was first discovered in 1943 in children born in the 1930s. Since then, it has increased worldwide.[205] The increase of autism has been linked to the increase in mercury exposure through fish and industrial sources, amalgam,[206] and additionally through increased parenteral exposure to ethylmercury thiosalicylate (thimerosal), first introduced by Eli Lilly and Company in the 1930s as a preservative in vaccinations.[207] In 1982, an expert panel at the FDA reviewed thimerosal and called for its removal in over-the-counter products. The panel reported that thimerosal was "toxic, caused cell damage, was not effective in killing bacteria or halting their replication" and was "not generally recognized as being safe or effective."[208] In 1991, senior executives of Merck were concerned that infants were getting too much mercury. The March 1991 memo, obtained by the Los Angeles Times (obtained well over a decade later published a piece in February 8, 2005), said that six-month-old children who received shots on schedule would get a mercury dose eighty-seven times higher than the maximum daily consumption guideline of mercury from fish. "The mercury load appears rather large," said the memo from Maurice R. Hilleman written to the president of Merck's vaccine division. "The key issue is whether Thimerosal, in the amount given with the vaccine, does or does not constitute a safety hazard." (He retired as a senior VP at Merck in 1984.)

In 1988, the FDA ruled that thimerosal be removed from OTC products but gave the industry another sixteen years to phase out thimerosal's use. In 1999, the FDA stated that mercury exposure from vaccines exceeded Federal Safety Guidelines. On November 15, 1999, the FDA nominated thimerosal to the Center for the Evaluation of Risks to Human Reproduction, and on at least two occasions the core Scientific Advisory Board recommended further evaluation. This triggered a panic in 1999 among the Public Health Service (PHS) and the American Academy of Pediatrics (AAP), as they were anticipating public outrage (that never came); nevertheless, they first announced that thimerosal should be removed from vaccines:

> Because any potential risk is of concern, the Public Health Service (PHS), the American Academy of Pediatrics (AAP), and vaccine manufacturers agree that Thimerosal-containing vaccines should be removed as soon as possible.
>
> Similar conclusions were reached this year in a meeting attended by European regulatory agencies, European vaccine manufacturers, and FDA, which examined the use of Thimerosal-containing vaccines produced or sold in European countries.[209]

The prevalence of autism in the United States became epidemic (an increase of 5 in 10,000 to 60 in 10,000) when additional thimerosal-containing vaccines were introduced for newborns in the early 1990s. Newborns up to the age of six months began to be regularly exposed to a cumulative thimerosal dose of 187.5 µg.[210] At the same time, most other countries, such as Germany and Denmark, where thimerosal doses were reduced, reported much lower autism prevalence.

Now, as has been frequently pointed out, "it" is never just one thing, but mercury is a toxic linchpin when it comes to many neurodegenerative disorders and is certainly synergistic with other toxins, such as glyphosate.

At the end of 2015 it was announced that the rate of autism was now 1 in 45, but authorities have reassured us that today's doctors and parents are just so much better at recognizing autism then we were thirty years ago when the rate was 1 in 10,000. But the sad truth is that if officialdom ever acknowledged there was a real increase that was not just due to better awareness or diagnosis, then they would have to address the cause.

Nothing is wrong, keep calm, and pay no attention to all these children who were always there but not seen or talked about. This is the propaganda that must be pushed, for as long as the public at large buys that, then issues related to thimerosol and vaccines and the pesticides in our environment can remain a mere academic argument.

Well. If these children have always been here, then where are the official government statistics showing all the autistic adults we were somehow blind to?

The medical community has really failed big time on this one, so convinced are they that all this autism is because doctors are smarter than they used to be. I hope I am smarter than I used to be when the rates were 1 in 10,000, but I was not so dumb in the 1980s to miss all these affected children—they just were not there. I never saw one child with autism in medical school or during my pediatric residency in Los Angeles—never even heard of any physician seeing one. I didn't see my first patient with what I believed was autism until 1989.

The children with autism are just the canaries in the proverbial coal mine. The health of all children in the United States is disintegrating while we pretend that there is nothing to be concerned about.

## TRACE AMOUNTS

Bertrand Russell in the *The Impact of Science on Society* (1953, p. 50) said, "Diet, injections, and injunctions will combine, from a very early age, to produce the sort of character and the sort of beliefs that the authorities consider desirable, and any serious criticism of the powers that be will become psychologically impossible. Even if all are miserable, all will believe themselves happy, because the government will tell them that they are so."

In the United States today, the mercury present in vaccines has supposedly been reduced to trace amounts (if you can trust the vaccine manufacturers' word for this, which one can't), except in the majority of flu vaccines. So, why does the autism rate keep on going up?

At the end of this chapter, you will read my resignation letter to the American Academy of Pediatrics wherein I explained just how toxic even trace amounts of mercury are, and again how the vaccine industry can't be trusted to tell the truth about any of the ingredients or the amounts of any ingredient in their vaccines.

Who knows how much mercury is actually in some of these vaccines even today?

The study that concerned the CDC in 2000 showed that post-vaccination mercury levels were significantly higher in preterm infants compared with term infants in regard to the hepatitis B injections at birth.[211] The concern appeared to be not about the impact mercury could have on newborns but on the impact it could have on the vaccination compliance rates. To mitigate any problems the Stajich study might have, or if word leaked out about the then-embargoed Verstraeten data[212] (showing a direct link between thimerosal and the epidemic of neurodevelopmental disorders, including autism), the CDC contracted with Dr. Pichichero, an academician in their control, to undertake a study similar to Dr. Stajich's but to produce different results.

The results of this alliance between the CDC/NIP officials and Pichichero at the University of Rochester resulted in what was hoped would be the definitive thimerosal study[213] to prove that thimerosal was not toxic in amounts found in childhood vaccines. A number of governmental committees (CDC, FDA, etc.), of which vaccine manufacturer employees were members, formed to review the problem as well.[214] Verstraeten (CDC/GlaxoSmithKline) diluted Pichichero's original epidemiological study to show that there was no causation between thimerosal and autism or any other neurodevelopmental problem.[215]

Perhaps this is a good place to introduce Dr. William Thompson, the CDC whistle-blower who came forward in 2014. Thompson admitted that the CDC had deliberately withheld crucial evidence proving that the MMR (measles, mumps, and rubella) vaccine caused autism. It is true that the MMR has no mercury in it, but when you are already poisoned with mercury and pesticides, the vaccine itself (contaminated with cancer-causing avian retrovirus) doesn't need to have mercury in it.

Dr. Thompson revealed that when African-American boys under the age of thirty-six months were given the MMR vaccine, the rate of autism in this group rose by almost 400 percent (see statement below).

The CDC solved this nightmare by eliminating from the data all African-American boys without a Georgia birth certificate. It is called fudging the data to get the results you want. They could have just as easily pulled all black males from the study who did not have a valid driver's license. Yes, toddlers never have driver's licenses—that is the point. The sample size was reduced 41 percent, and the statistical significance of the finding vanished.

On August 27, 2014, William Thompson, PhD, issued this statement:

FOR IMMEDIATE RELEASE—AUGUST 27, 2014 STATEMENT OF WILLIAM W. THOMPSON, Ph.D., REGARDING THE 2004 ARTICLE EXAMINING THE POSSIBILITY OF A RELATIONSHIP BETWEEN MMR VACCINE AND AUTISM

My name is William Thompson. I am a Senior Scientist with the Centers for Disease Control and Prevention, where I have worked since 1998.

I regret that my co-authors and I omitted statistically significant information in our 2004 article published in the journal *Pediatrics*. The omitted data suggested that African American males who received the MMR vaccine before age thirty-six months were at increased risk for autism.

Decisions were made regarding which findings to report after the data were collected, and I believe that the final study protocol was not followed.

I want to be absolutely clear that I believe vaccines have saved and continue to save countless lives. I would never suggest that any parent avoid vaccinating children of any race. Vaccines prevent serious diseases, and the risks associated with their administration are vastly outweighed by their individual and societal benefits.

My concern has been the decision to omit relevant findings in a particular study for a particular sub group for a particular vaccine. There have always been recognized risks for vaccination and I believe it is the responsibility of the CDC to properly convey the risks associated with receipt of those vaccines.[216]

Dr. Thompson also revealed that not only had the MMR been responsible for an increase in the cases of autism seen in African-American boys, but that vaccinating pregnant women with vaccinations containing thimerosal is known to cause children to suffer from tics (sudden, repetitive movements or sounds that can be difficult to control): "Thimerosal from vaccines causes tics. You start a campaign and make it your mantra. Do you think a pregnant mother would want to take a vaccine that they knew caused tics? Absolutely not, I would never give my wife a vaccine that I thought caused tics. I can say tics are four times more prevalent in kids with autism. There is a biological plausibility right now to say that thimerosal causes autism like features!"[217]

Verstraeten diluted this data several times until all significance had vanished and then "lost" all the data so it could not be reviewed. J. Codero, assistant surgeon general and director of the National Center on Birth Defects and Developmental Disabilities, attached a cover letter to a manuscript that was eventually published as "Thimerosal and the occurrence of autism: negative ecological evidence from Danish population-based data." Codero and others wanted to make sure the misleading study was published.

The Danish population studies, as they became known, were authored by the Office of the Inspector General (OIG) fugitive Poul Thorsen, who is now one of OIG's Most Wanted. The CDC was paying him to write fraudulent studies for them making the medical community think there is no link between vaccines and autism. He didn't have to steal money—he was already stealing money. The million he took was a payoff almost any way you look at it.

This is from the OIG website:

- From approximately February 2004 until February 2010, Poul Thorsen executed a scheme to steal grant money awarded by the Centers for Disease Control and Prevention (CDC). CDC had awarded grant money to Denmark for research involving infant disabilities, autism, genetic disorders, and fetal alcohol syndrome. CDC awarded the grant to fund studies of the relationship between autism and the exposure to vaccines, the relationship between cerebral palsy and infection during pregnancy, and the relationship between developmental outcomes and fetal alcohol exposure.

- Thorsen worked as a visiting scientist at CDC, Division of Birth Defects and Developmental Disabilities, before the grant was awarded.
- The initial grant was awarded to the Danish Medical Research Council. In approximately 2007, a second grant was awarded to the Danish Agency for Science, Technology, and Innovation. Both agencies are governmental agencies in Denmark. The research was done by the Aarhaus University and Odense University Hospital in Denmark.
- Thorsen allegedly diverted over $1 million of the CDC grant money to his own personal bank account. Thorsen submitted fraudulent invoices on CDC letterhead to medical facilities assisting in the research for reimbursement of work allegedly covered by the grants. The invoices were addressed to Aarhaus University and Sahlgrenska University Hospital. The fact that the invoices were on CDC letterhead made it appear that CDC was requesting the money from Aarhaus University and Sahlgrenska University Hospital, although the bank account listed on the invoices belonged to Thorsen.
- In April 2011, Thorsen was indicted on 22 counts of Wire Fraud and Money Laundering.
- According to bank account records, Thorsen purchased a home in Atlanta, a Harley Davidson motorcycle, an Audi automobile, and a Honda SUV with funds that he received from the CDC grants.
- Thorsen is currently in Denmark and is awaiting extradition to the United States.[218]

This is from the OIG website of their most-wanted fugitives, which makes it sound like Thorsen was under arrest—only some paperwork was needed—before he was shipped off to the United States.[219] But the truth is that the million he stole was just as likely a payoff for writing up the faux scientific papers the CDC wanted him to write.

The OIG statement that Thorsen is awaiting extradition is pure doublespeak. Today, Thorsen is engaging in his normal routine activities, including his academic career. He goes to conferences, such as in the UK—don't expect him to be arrested or detained. No one in the government wants him to tell his story in a court of law. He would spill the beans on the corruption at the CDC. He is even still publishing papers.[220] "Stealing" a cool million sounds more like a payoff than an unsanctioned crime in light of the lack of effort in extraditing or arresting him and the fact he continues life as normal. He didn't even have to fake his death like some others have done.

## VACCINE SAFETY DATA

The CDC has assembled the vaccine safety data link (VSDL), which includes the medical records of 9 million vaccinated children and the precise vaccines they received and at what ages. The CDC used the data link to do the original Verstratten "Generation Zero" study in 2000 and found a 1,160 percent relative risk for children exposed to 26 µg or more of thimerosol compared those exposed to 25 µg or less. Afterwards, the agency transferred the VSDL to a private insurance company, the American Health Insurance Plan (AHIP), to protect the data from ever being studied by independent scientists. The CDC can now say that the private company to which it entrusted the federal data is not subject to the federal Freedom of Information Act.

In 2001, the CDC and its Office of the National Immunization Program also contracted with the Institute of Medicine (IOM) to create the Immunization Safety Review Committee (ISRC), presumably for damage control against the mounting thimerosal vaccine injury evidence.[221] The IOM's first report on thimerosal was issued in October of 2001.[222] "[The CDC] wants us to declare, well, these things are pretty safe on a population basis," stated Dr. Marie McCormick, chairman of the ISRC. This committee met to address the question of whether exposure to thimerosal-containing vaccines could be associated with adverse neurodevelopmental disorders, and the committee stated they found the hypothesis "biologically plausible." They had different marching orders despite being told, "We said this before you got here, and I think we said this yesterday, the point of no return, the line we will not cross in public policy is to pull the vaccine, change the schedule. We could say it is time to revisit this, but we would never recommend that level. Even recommending research is recommendations for policy. We wouldn't say compensate, we wouldn't say pull the vaccine, we wouldn't say stop the program" by Kathleen Stratton, PhD, IOM staff and study director, ISRC. "We are not ever going to come down that it[223] is a true side effect," said McCormick, even before the IOM had considered any evidence.

Nevertheless, the IOM committee concluded, "The committee recommends that full consideration be given by appropriate professional societies and governmental agencies to removing thimerosal from vaccines administered to infants, children, or pregnant women in the United States." The CDC called the IOM committee to meet again in 2004 after it was made clear they would reach the unequivocal conclusion that there is no causality between vaccines and autism or any other neurological injury. The IOM would base its final conclusions on epidemiological research already proven to be flawed or fabricated and authored by Thorsen—one of the OIG's Most Wanted.

The IOM ignored anything that was not aligned with its orders from the CDC; no evidence was embraced that was in conflict with CDC vaccine recommendations. On May 18, 2004, the IOM's ISRC issued their final report, which found the body of epidemiological evidence favored a rejection of a causal relationship between exposure to the vaccine thimerosal and autism. In the years since it was issued, the IOM report has been successfully used to silence media inquiries into vaccine safety, as a defense for ignoring thousands upon thousands of petitions for repressing information about vaccine injuries in the federal vaccine court, as justification for eliminating federal funding on research of the vaccine/autism link, and as justification for the federal preemption of vaccine control and the push to eliminate parental exemptions.

The FDA has never ordered the recall of mercury-laden vaccines, which continued to be used almost exclusively through 2002 and 2003. In 2005, when it appeared that autism rates were starting to decrease coincident with the removal of thimerosal from the vaccines in the routine schedule,[224] the CDC significantly broadened its flu-shot recommendations, so that by the age of five years, children exposed to an all-thimerosal schedule of flu shots would get 53 percent of the mercury children received from all shots in 1999. The additional recommendation to vaccine pregnant women would only add to the mercury burden. If this was done on purpose, to obfuscate the falling autism rates, there was a reason, as you will read.

The World Health Organization Strategic Group of Experts (SAGE) met in June of 2001 and stated their objective clearly: "WHO was extremely anxious to preserve the production of vaccines. Industry is expecting clear signals from WHO on the Thimerosal issue, and has been confirmed by informal consultations with some manufacturers during the first half of 2001." At WHO headquarters in Geneva, a meeting was held on May 21, 2002, titled "WHO Informal Meeting on Removal of Thimerosal from Vaccines and Its Implications for Global Vaccine Supply." From the meeting summary, more objectives were enumerated, such as

(1) Obtaining regulatory approval for the new formulated Thimerosal reduced or removed vaccines involves complex activities that are costly and time-consuming; (2) WHO is concerned about the current situation whereby manufacturers in developed countries have been forced to lower the Thimerosal content of their vaccines; (3) The option of using single dose vaccines is not feasible for WHO . . . upgrading the infrastructure would result in huge increase in vaccine cost.

The meeting memo went on to state, "In view of the situation, WHO is faced with . . . support maintenance of Thimerosal as an effective preservative in multidose and possibly also in single dose vaccines." Lastly, the memo stated, "The actions required from WHO in order to ensure continued availability of these vaccines include the following: Develop a strong advocacy campaign to support ongoing use of Thimerosal."

In other words, agencies outside of the United States, such as WHO,[225] the Global Alliance for Vaccines and Immunization (GAVI), and the International Brighton Collaboration, seem to be having untoward influence on vaccine policy inside the United States. This influence apparently brought the thimerosal-laden flu vaccine into the routine vaccine schedule years after the AAP recommended the elimination of thimerosal. Since WHO will not use any multidose vaccine that is not licensed in the United States, and it insists on using multidose vaccines, it therefore must keep the uses of vaccine viable in the United States.

This mercury problem would be solved if a vaccine maker substituted a non-thimerosal preservative, but that would require them to submit a new drug application, even though only the preservative has changed. The fee that must be paid to the FDA for each new application is in the millions. One solution would be to have Congress request that the FDA waive the fee for the purpose of removing thimerosal from a biologic/vaccine. This would be the logical approach, but obfuscation seems to rule the day. In the meantime, developmental (behavioral) disorders have increased to one out of every six children in the United States.

They say truth is stranger than fiction, and the truth is WHO, the UN, the CDC, etc., don't care if there is something toxic in vaccines because they mean to do harm.

Really . . . harm? Ask why would "they" want to give the flu vaccine to pregnant women, for example. They will say it is because getting the flu while you are pregnant can injure the baby. While there is some truth to that, it is the cytokine storm the immune system kicks up that could injure the baby—not the virus itself. But guess what the flu vaccine causes? Yep, a cytokine storm!

So, what is the deal—why all the push for vaccines for everything without informed consent?

Vaccines have been used secretly to sterilize women of child-bearing age in order to test the efficacy of using a vaccine as a means for population control.

Vaccines are not only big, no-risk moneymakers, but they are the sacred-cow tool eugenicists plan to utilize for their population-control agendas. That is why they can't be criticized for any reason. The population must be willing to take vaccines for this plan to work.

Vaccines have essentially become a soft-kill bioweapon.

In 2014, Kenya's Catholic bishops charged two United Nations organizations with sterilizing millions of girls and women under cover of an anti-tetanus inoculation program sponsored by the Kenyan government.

The Kenya Catholic Doctors Association found an antigen that causes miscarriages in a vaccine being administered to 2.3 million girls and women by WHO and UNICEF. The vaccines were all laced with hCG—human chorionic gonadatropin.

Dr. Ngare, spokesman for the Kenya Catholic Doctors Association, stated in a bulletin released November 4, 2014, "This proved right our worst fears; that this WHO campaign is not about eradicating neonatal tetanus but a well-coordinated forceful population control mass sterilization exercise using a proven fertility regulating vaccine. This evidence was presented to the Ministry of Health before the third round of immunization but was ignored."[226]

So, what happened?

Dr. Ngare,[227] who had warned that the Kenyan government might skew joint tests with samples that did not come from the suspected WHO campaign, now says that is just what happened. "The normal vaccine used in hospitals is not the problem. People can take that safely."

The Kenyan government was supposed to use an equal number of samples from the bishops and the government, but when three of the resulting 19 samples proved positive for HCG, the government submitted another 40 samples, also from their stores. "The results of these 40 vials were loaded onto the previously completed results of 19 vials from the joint committee," claim the bishops. "This was aimed at creating a dilution and bias of the 3 vials that were positive out of 9." [228]

So, nothing to see here . . . move along.

The public is not supposed to know vaccines are being used as depopulation weapons. Depopulation is designed to get rid of large numbers of people who might interfere with globalist interests in taking control of resources, and they produce lots of greenhouse gas.

In November 1993, the *FASEB* Journal (volume 7, pp. 1381–85) published an article that said, "Our study provides insights into possible modes of action of the birth control vaccine promoted by the Task Force on Birth Control Vaccines of the WHO (World Health Organization)."

An article in the *British Medical Bulletin* (volume 49, 1993), "Contraceptive Vaccines," states:

Three major approaches to contraceptive vaccine development are being pursued at the present time. The most advanced approach, which has already reached the stage of phase 2 clinical trials, involves the induction of immunity against human chorionic gonadotropin (hCG). Vaccines are being engineered . . . incorporating tetanus or diphtheria toxoid linked to a variety of hCG-based peptides. . . . Clinical trials have revealed that such preparations are capable of stimulating the production of anti-hCG antibodies.

The fundamental principle behind this approach to contraceptive vaccine development is to prevent the maternal recognition of pregnancy by inducing a state of immunity against hGC, the hormone that signals the presence of the embryo to the maternal endocrine system.

In principle, the induction of immunity against hGC should lead to a sequence of normal, or slightly extended, menstrual cycles during which any pregnancies would be terminated.

During the next decade the world's population is set to rise by around 500 million. Moreover, because the rates of population growth in the developing countries of Africa, South America, and Asia will be so much greater than the rest of the world, the distribution of this dramatic population growth will be uneven.

The diphtheria and tetanus vaccines would function as a social and political mask to hide the sterilizing intent as millions of women in the Third World receive vaccines they're told would protect them against infections and disease.

In a letter to the medical journal the *Lancet* titled "Cameroon: Vaccination and Politics," Peter Ndumbe and Emmanuel Yenshu, the authors of this letter, report on their efforts to analyze widespread popular resistance to a tetanus vaccine given in the northwest province of Cameroon. Two of the reasons women rejected the vaccine: it was given only to "females of childbearing age," and people heard that a "sterilizing agent" was present in the vaccine.[229] The reason they heard there was such an agent is that there was!

The well-known journalist Alexander Cockburn, who passed in 2012, wrote on the op-ed page of the *LA Times* on September 8, 1994, an article titled "Real U.S. Policy in Third World: Sterilization: Disregard the 'Empowerment' Shoe Polish—the goal is to keep the natives from breeding." In the article, he reviewed the infamous Kissinger-commissioned 1974 National Security Study Memorandum 200, "which addressed population issues":

The true concern of Kissinger analysts [in Memorandum 200] was maintenance of US access to Third World resources. They worried that the "political consequences" of population growth [in the Third World] could produce internal instability. . . . With famine and food riots and the breakdown of social order in such countries, [the Kissinger memo warns that] "the smooth flow of needed materials will be jeopardized.

In other words, too many people equal disruption for the transnational corporations, whose intent is to steal resources from the people who live in various nations.

Cockburn noted that the writers of the Kissinger memo "favored sterilization over food aid." He goes on to say, "By 1977, Reimart Ravenholt, the director of AID's [US Agency for International Development] population program, was saying that his Agency's goal was to sterilize one-quarter of the world's women."

Tetanus vaccine protocols indicate that one injection is good for ten years. Therefore, multiple injections would indicate another motive for the vaccinations—such as the anti-fertility effect of hCG planted in the vaccine.

The Population Research Institute, in the November/December 1996 issue of its *Review,* published a report by David Morrison in which he states:

> Philippine women may have been unwittingly vaccinated against their own children, a recent study conducted by the Philippine Medical Association (PMA) has indicated.
>
> The study tested random samples of a tetanus vaccine for the presence of human chorionic gonadotropin (hCG), a hormone essential to the establishment and maintenance of pregnancy. . . . The PMA's positive test results indicate that just such an abortifacient may have been administered to Philippine women without their consent.
>
> The PMA notified the Philippine Department of Health (PDOH) of these findings in a 16 September letter signed by the researchers and certified by its President. Using an immunological assay developed by the Food and Drug Administration in the United States, a three-doctor research panel tested forty-seven vials of tetanus vaccine collected at random from various health centers in Luzon and Mindanao. Nine were found to contain hCG in levels ranging from 0.191680 mIU/ml to 3.046061 mIU/ml. These vaccines, most of which were labeled as of Canadian origin, were supplied by the World Health Organization as part of a WHO-sponsored [sterilization] vaccination program.

Morrison's article implied that the vials of vaccine tested came from a widespread immunization campaign rather than from a small pilot study of a few women.

The Task Force on Vaccines for Fertility Regulation was created at the World Health Organization in 1973. Ute Sprenger, writing in *Biotechnology and Development Monitor* (December 1995) describes the task force as "a global coordinating body for anti-fertility vaccine R&D . . . such as anti-sperm and anti-ovum vaccines and vaccines designed to neutralize the biological functions of hCG."

Sprenger indicates that as of 1995, there were several large groups research-ing these vaccines. Among them:

- WHO/HRP. HRP is the Special Progamme of Research, Development and Research Training in Human Reproduction, located in Switzerland. It is funded by "the governments of Sweden, United Kingdom, Norway, Denmark, Germany and Canada, as well as the UNFPA and the World Bank."
- The Population Council, a US group funded by the Rockefeller Founda-tion, the National Institutes of Health (a US federal agency), and the US Agency for International Development (notorious for its collaborations with the CIA).
- National Institute of Immunology, located in India. "Major funders are the Indian government, the Canadian International Development Research Center and the (ubiquitous) Rockefeller Foundation."
- The Center for Population Research, located at the US National Insti-tute of Child Health and Development, which is part of the US National Institutes of Health.

The *Lancet* (4 June, 1998, p. 1272) stated, "During the recent National Immunisa-tion Campaign (vaccination for childhood diseases and tetanus toxoid for preg-nant women), in some villages [of Thailand] the women escaped and hid in the bushes thinking that they were going to be given injections to stop them having children."

AP, *Boston Globe* (October 10, 1992) published an article, "Birth-Control Vac-cine Is Reported in India," part of which reads, "Scientists said yesterday they have created the first birth-control shot for women, effective for an entire year . . . [after which] a booster shot is needed."

The point of all this is that vaccines have become a tool for depopulation, and that fact alone explains both the irrational overuse of them on the population and why they have been elevated to the status of a sacred cow where no untoward word can be said about their efficacy or safety. And those who make them are immune from liability.

West Nile, SARS, bird flu, swine flu, Ebola, Zika . . . *what is the real reason* for promoting these "epidemics"? To motivate populations to take the post-epi-demic vaccines that have undisclosed properties. Post COVID we now know the Spike protein that the modified mRNA bioweapon had the human body make has a special affinity for ovaries and testes. We have not seen the worst yet from this bioweapon be it from sterilization or turbo-cancers.

*Never* lose the right to exempt yourself or your children from taking a vaccine—*never lose this right*! Once this right is lost, a public health police state will be here.

# AMALGAM

*"Those who can get you to believe absurdities can get you to commit atrocities."*

—Voltaire

In 1830, amalgam fillings were first used in the United States. By 1840, organized dentistry denounced the use of amalgam as a poor filling material due to concerns about mercury poisoning. The American Society of Dental Surgeons was formed and required members to sign a pledge promising not to use mercury fillings. The American Dental Association was formed in 1859 by those dentists who supported the use of mercury amalgam as the filling material of choice, which it still supports today.

In 1926, a chemist, Dr. Alfred Stock, noted that mercury amalgam fillings in the mouth were a source of mercury vapor.[230] Fifty years later, the FDA pronounced acceptance of amalgam fillings and grandfathered their approval under the GRAS (generally recognized as safe) category due to its long-term usage. It has never budged from that position. Amalgam fillings have been shown to be a source of mercury nephrotoxicity as demonstrated by Boyd et al.[231] in an animal model, and by Mortada et al.[232] in 101 humans. Animal and in vitro studies have shown that exposure to inorganic and metallic mercury causes neuronal damage[233] and biochemical alterations (inclusive induction of β-amyloid) found in Alzheimer's disease,[234] even at very low levels (where other metals like Al, Cd, Pb, Mn, Zn, Fe, Cr, and Cu were not able to cause this type of neuronal alterations).

Mercury levels in human placentas correlate with the number of maternal amalgam fillings, and a substantial amount of mercury from amalgam reaches the fetus.[235] Mercury from dental amalgam in pregnant women was reported by Holmes to contribute to the development of autism in their children.[236] In this study mothers of ninety-four autistic children had statistically more amalgam fillings during pregnancy than forty-nine mothers of normal controls. In contrast to their higher mercury exposure during pregnancy, these autistic children had reduced mercury levels in their first haircut, reflecting a reduced capacity to excrete mercury from their body, which in turn may lead to elevated brain mercury levels.

It is interesting to compare this study to that of Grandjean et al., who found that infants who reached milestone criteria early had significantly higher mercury concentrations in the hair at twelve months of age.[237] This is completely consistent with Holmes's finding: the ability to excrete mercury (high hair levels of mercury) is clearly neuroprotective, and an inability to excrete mercury (low hair levels) is not neuroprotective. The neurobehavioral effects resulting from exposure to low levels of mercury from dental amalgam have been described.[238] Low-dose exposure to inorganic mercury may be a cofactor in the development of autoimmune diseases as well[239]—a finding that has been duplicated by other researchers.[240]

The CDC took funding from thimerosal research, based on the 2004 IOM recommendations that were predetermined by the CDC to fit their pro-mercury agenda, and then threatened those who held and sought NIH grants to drop their current thimerosal research and have no further involvement in thimerosal research.[241]

Today, we know that the CDC and their contractors intentionally fabricated research, suppressed data, and lied to the American people and the world.

Berlin suggested that the frequency of pathological side effects from amalgam due to a genetically determined susceptibility is about 1 percent.[242] The German Commission on Human Biological Monitoring states that genetically susceptible individuals may develop immune-mediated responses to amalgam. The portion of persons in the general public is about 1 percent to 4 percent.[243] Richardson concludes that approximately 20 percent of the general public may experience subclinical central nervous system and/or kidney function impairment due to amalgam fillings.[244]

Mercury can be exported from the United States only if it is for medical or dental purposes. The motivation to protect mercury amalgam material is fueled by the fact that there may now be as many as 20 million illegal gold-prospecting operations going on in sixty countries.

## US-SIGNED TREATY "UPHOLDS USE OF AMALGAM".

On November 14, 2013, the association commended public health provisions in a global mercury treaty that "upholds the use of dental amalgam, a durable, safe, effective cavity-filling material." The United States signed and offered acceptance documents November 6, joining other nations in moving the legally binding treaty forward.

A Department of State official signed the Minamata Convention on Mercury and deposited the US Instrument of Acceptance to enable the United States to become a party to the convention, said a media note at the department's website. The Minamata Convention was concluded by the United States as an executive agreement, and a State Department official told the ADA News no further congressional action is required.

Now, dental supply companies are free to ship the most nonradioactive toxic element to illegal gold-mining operations that are devastating the environment in South America and other locations.

This is an important environmental issue, but exposing the various dental supply companies in the United States and their ties to the ADA is beyond the scope of this book. If you need any proof that this is taking place under everyone's nose, then read this little blurb from a 2007 US Geological Survey:

> Site visits were made to dental supply stores in Lima, a dental clinic at the Universidad Cayetano Heredia in Lima, and to a dental office in Trujillo. Bulk mercury in 100-g plastic bottles is sold in the dental supply stores in the 200 block of Avenida Emancipación in Lima. Several gold shops are nearby. Mercury sold in the dental supply shops is triple-distilled, has a label indicating that it has U.S. Food and Drug Administration approval, is imported from the United States, and distributed by a Peruvian importer. The cost is approximately $7 (S/.22) for the 100-g bottle, and no professional documentation is needed for purchase.[245]

There is no question that mercury exported from the United States, supposedly for dental fillings, is being used for purposes other than dental fillings, but the practice requires that the use of mercury dental amalgam continue to be allowed in the United States.

## EFFICACY AND SAFETY?

In the early twentieth century, the epidemic of acrodynia (pink disease) affected up to 1 in 500 infants in some industrial countries until teething powders which contained mercury as calomel ($Hg_2Cl_2$) was removed from the market. Calomel, when given orally, is about 100-fold less toxic than ethylmercury (thimerosal) to neurons in vitro[246] and poisons the nerves in the baby's gums.[247]

Once calomel was removed from the market, acrodynia fell below the clinicians' radar, although it started to affect children again in the 1990s when there were so many vaccines loaded with the full complement of thimerosal. But the often mild, self-limiting, exfoliating rash on the hands of children was not recognized as a reaction to the mercury in vaccines. No controlled, randomized study regarding the safety of amalgam or thimerosal exists, yet these exposures seem to be crucial in the pathogenesis of autism. Furthermore, there are no studies comparing the health of individuals pre- or post-exposure or exposure versus non-exposure.

In Minamata, a single corporation was able to obfuscate the damage they were causing with mercury for decades, but the situation with the mercury in biologics is much more pernicious. The FDA, NIH, and CDC seem to have been unduly influenced by vaccine manufacturers or dental boards and even seem to share co-employees thereof.[248] Why have thimerosal and dental amalgam, both of which consist of about 50 percent of the most toxic nonradioactive element known, been allowed to bypass toxicological testing?

As with thimerosal, the literature on amalgam toxicity[249] is used inappropriately to attest to its harmlessness.[250] The effort being expended to keep mercury biologics in use is about money, but few are the dentists or the physicians who will have an awareness of why they were brainwashed to defend this most toxic element.

In July of 2015, it was revealed[251] that the Department of Health and Human Services squelched the FDA proposal that would have limited dentists' use of mercury. Approved by the FDA in late 2011 and kept secret since, the proposal would have advised dentists not to use mercury fillings in cavities in pregnant women, nursing moms, children under six years old, and people with mercury allergies, kidney diseases, or neurological problems.

It also urged dentists to avoid using fillings that contain mercury compounds in any patient, where possible.

So much for transparency in government. HHS said it would cost too much—bet they didn't figure in the cost of the disease and suffering mercury causes!

## THE BIOCHEMISTRY OF MERCURY EXPOSURE

Representing the American Academy of Pediatrics at the Simpsonwood meeting in June 2000, Bill Weil, MD, said, "There are just a host of neurodevelopmental data that would suggest that we've got a serious problem. . . . To think there isn't some possible problem here is unreal."

Ethylmercury is not safer mercury than methylmercury. When most physicians try to defend ethylmercury, they say the concern is about methylmercury not ethyl-, so thimerosal is not a deep concern: "Why, it is no worse than eating a tuna sandwich." Now, there are quacks (literally) who will think and say this, but because of the apparent disinformation surrounding thimerosal, it is worth noting what toxicologists have understood for the last few decades regarding the comparative toxicology of ethyl- and methylmercury:[252] "There was little difference in the neurotoxicities of methyl mercury and ethyl mercury when effects on the dorsal root ganglia or coordination disorders were compared." Further, "the neurological signs and symptoms of methyl and ethyl mercury intoxication are identical."

Unlike the quacks, who will not show you anything other than their own fudged science in an insane effort to defend quackery, there is actually a lot of science, and while it is somewhat dry, a fraction is included here because it needs to be on the record.

A recent study using infant *Macaca fascicularis* primates exposed to injected ethylmercury and those exposed to equal amounts of ingested methylmercury showed that those injected with ethylmercury retained twice as much inorganic mercury in their brains in comparison to the methylmercury-exposed primates.[253] These primates were exposed to mercury levels at a rate equal to what children in the United States received via standard childhood vaccines from 1991 to 2003.

The Environmental Protection Agency considers any material that has greater than 200 ppb of mercury to be hazardous waste. A thimerosal vaccine (1:10000 thimerosal) exceeds this value by 250 times, or 50,000 ppb mercury. A developing fetus would receive a dose of mercury that exceeds the federal limits by several hundred-fold when the mother is injected with a thimerosal-containing vaccine. Furthermore, fetal blood mercury concentrations have been shown to be as much as 4.4 times greater than in maternal blood,[254] which would result in an even greater relative distribution to the fetus.

In other words, the developing fetus acts as a mercury sink for its mother. Cysteine and glutathione synthesis are crucial for mercury detoxification, which is reduced in autistic children, possibly due to genetic polymorphisms.[255] Therefore, autistic children have 20 percent lower levels of cysteine and 54 percent lower levels of glutathione, which adversely affect their ability to detoxify and excrete metals like mercury.[256] This leads to a higher concentration of free mercury in blood, which then transfers into tissues and increases the half-life of mercury in the body, as compared to children with normal levels of cysteine and glutathione.

As was shown by Bradstreet et al. in a study involving 221 autistic children, vaccinated autistic children showed an elevation of urinary mercury about six-fold higher than normal controls after appropriate mobilization with the chelating agent DMSA.[257] Delayed detoxification of mercury severely impairs methylation reactions (required for the correct expression of DNA, RNA, and neurotransmitters), which further adversely affects growth-factor-derived development of the brain and attention abilities. Phospholipid methylation, which is crucial for attention, is impaired in autistic and attention deficit hyperactivity disorders. Ethylmercury levels, seen ten days after vaccination with thimerosal doses lower than what infants received during the 1990s, produced greater than 50 percent inhibition of methylation. In vitro studies have shown that thimerosal was more than a hundred-fold more potent than inorganic mercury in inhibiting such essential methylation reactions. Inorganic mercury was found to be ten-fold more potent than lead in inhibition of neuronal microtubule.[258]

Inorganic mercury also leads to growth inhibition and denudation of neuronal growth cones. This was seen only fifteen minutes after exposure to very low levels of inorganic mercury, levels that were about 100- to 1,000-fold lower than found in brains of individuals with dental amalgam or Alzheimer's disease.[259]

It was also shown that concentrations of thimerosal, which can occur after vaccination, induce membrane and DNA damage and initiate apoptosis in human neurons.[260] Genotoxic effects were also observed in another in vitro study.[261] Autistic children seem to be genetically more susceptible to toxin-derived inhibition of methylation processes. It has been estimated that up to 15 percent of the population may show enhanced susceptibility to mercury exposure. Pichichero et al. "argued" that ethylmercury administered through vaccines is eliminated rapidly from the blood and rapidly excreted in stool, but only thirty-three children at the age of two and six months were used for blood mercury assessment, thus overlooking individuals with impaired mercury excretion. Furthermore, blood levels were obtained days to weeks after vaccination. Thus peak levels were not measured, and the thimerosal dose was much lower than that given via vaccination in the 1990s. Furthermore, the stool was not examined to determine if that was where the mercury ended up. Nevertheless, the authors concluded, "This study gives comforting reassurance about the safety of ethyl mercury as a preservative in childhood vaccines." This study was heavily criticized, including the conflicts of interest it contained.[262] When you are getting paid to prove a point, you prove it by hook or by crook. It's money and screw the science.

Levels of ethylmercury found eight days after vaccination leads to 50 percent inhibition of methionine synthase (MS). Compounding this toxic sequela of thimerosal, neurons are unable to synthesize cysteine, the rate-limiting amino acid for glutathione synthesis.[263] Thus, neurons are most sensitive to mercury toxicity since glutathione is the major intracellular agent in mercury and heavy-metal detoxification. It is known that thimerosal and inorganic mercury depletes intracellular glutathione levels, which subsequently leads to oxidative stress, neuronal cytotoxicity, and death.[264] The toxic effects of ethylmercury appear to be essentially identical to those of methylmercury as indicated by James et al.

## AUTOIMMUNITY

Autoimmunity as a cause of autism—triggered by bacterial antigens, dietary peptides, and mercury—has been proposed,[265] as has an increased risk of multiple sclerosis from thimerosal-containing hepatitis B vaccines.[266] Autopsied brains of autistic children demonstrated chronic activation of microglia and astrocytes indicative of an autoimmune process.[267] Mercury is a potent inducer of haptene-mediated autoimmune reactions, especially when exposure is repetitive, which is the case in children exposed early to iatrogenic mercury during pregnancy (from amalgam) and then after birth in the form of vaccines. Most studies neglect the importance of repetitive mercury exposures for the induction of autoimmunity. One study found that in autoimmune-sensitive mouse strains, vaccinations with thimerosal in doses and timing equivalent to those of the pediatric immunization schedule of the United States in 2001 led to profound behavioral and neuropathologic disturbances comparable to those of autism, and in another study the autoimmune reaction persisted long after mercury could no longer be detected.[268]

These reactions were noted despite thimerosal doses lower than the ones given to newborns in the 1990s in the United States. It was also shown that the risk of thimerosal sensitization is increased in individuals with gene deletions of the glutathione S-transferases M1 and T1.[269] Mercury also increases cytotoxicity of glutamate, which has been described in many neurodegenerative diseases. In vitro studies suggest that the neurotoxicity of thimerosal is enhanced through neomycin and aluminum hydroxide (ingredients in vaccines) and testosterone, while estrogen decreases the toxic effects.[270]

Estrogen has been shown to decrease the toxicity of inorganic mercury, which may in part explain the 4-to-1 ratio of boys to girls in autism cases. Lead may play a synergistic pathogenetic role in neurodevelopment disorders and autism. A combination of lead and mercury resulted in an increase of toxicity in vitro.[271]

## EPIDEMIOLOGICAL OBFUSCATION

Whenever I tell a colleague that you can't use epidemiology to prove that sex causes pregnancy, they always seem surprised, but the answer is very simple. Epidemiology counts numbers without a lot of context—biosemiotics is not part of epidemiology. You can count the number of people having sex, but without an understanding of what intercourse does biologically, you can't prove sex results in pregnancy. The most polite way of saying it is probably that it allows for a lot of interpretation. But the truth is that it allows for manipulation of statistics to reveal just about whatever you want those statistics to reveal, as long as someone who is an expert in epidemiology doesn't look over your shoulder.

Epidemiological studies have been scientifically compromised; nevertheless, using data from the Vaccine Adverse Events Reporting System (VAERS), Vaccine Safety Data (VSD), Biological Surveillance Summaries of the CDC, and the US Department of Education datasets, researchers found a significant correlation between the risk of autism, mental retardation, speech disorders, and heart disease and the cumulative thimerosal dose given via injection, which far exceeds (11- to 150-fold) the EPA- and FDA-established maximum permissible levels for the daily oral ingestion of methylmercury.[272]

After the publication of this data, access to the VSD was restricted for independent scientists, as previously noted.

One of the infamous Danish studies, previously mentioned in relation to Poul Thorsen, actually claimed thimerosal protected children from autism. Those studies were as relevant as studying the effect of mosquitoes on the spread of malaria but doing the study in Minnesota versus Panama. The four published articles that are collectively known as the Danish Study[273] comprise a deliberate and coordinated effort to overshadow the emerging evidence connecting thimerosal to autism by a single network of authors almost all beholden to a single employer. This coordination involved individuals as high as the assistant surgeon general, J. Codero, as mentioned previously.

The four articles were based on a slightly different, but analytically non-comparable, view of the same overtly flawed data. The authors all had ties to a for-profit Danish vaccine manufacturer, the Statens Serum Institut (SSI), and this significant conflict of interest was not disclosed or reported in any of the journals that published the Danish Study. CDC employees and consultants were three of the seventeen authors. SSI directly employed six of the remaining fifteen authors, and SSI, through the Danish Epidemiology Science Centre, indirectly employed the remaining authors. SSI has a direct financial interest in the assessment of past thimerosal vaccine issues as well as in maintaining the continued viability of thimerosal-laden vaccines. These are the studies being referred to by those who keep repeating the mantra "vaccines are safe—the science is in."

## GARBAGE IN? GARBAGE OUT IS MORE ACCURATE

The US government is not the Chisso Corporation, but on many levels, from autism to AD, the government created its own variant of Minamata disease by using analogous denials, deceptions, governmental-corporate collusion, lack of accountability, and the arrogant continued use of mercury-laden biologics. The FDA panel in 1982 said thimerosal was "toxic, caused cell damage, was not effective in killing bacteria or halting their replication" and that thimerosal is "not generally recognized as being safe or effective."[274] Learning-disabled and autistic children are living the burden of proof. What happened? Where is the precautionary principle?

When something atrocious is done, there always seems to be the justification that it is preventing something even more atrocious. As the evidence continues to mount on what may be the largest iatrogenic public health disaster to affect this nation, so too does it appear that the apparent justification for deliberately letting this continue was about protecting the vaccine program's viability (or profitability). However, such rationalizations have propelled matters down a slippery slope. What little altruism there is in this justification belies individuals protecting careers, status, and reputations. This disaster did not come out of nowhere, and ultimately it will be found that it could have been mitigated if not for the irresponsible use of power and influence by an unholy alliance between corporation and state.

It also calls into question whether this public health fiasco was an isolated scenario. Mercury in biologics is a clear and present danger to the public health, and the only sane thing to do is end the obfuscation of an issue that may literally be destroying our society. Thimerosal has been banned in virtually all First World countries except the United States. And so the autism pandemic continues in the United States unabated.

A country of jobless and dependent learning-disabled and autistic children changes the United States as we know it. Ten years from now the United States may no longer be a First World country because of this. UC Davis health economists have for the first time projected the total costs of caring for all people with autism spectrum disorder, or ASD, in the United States for the current calendar year. Costs also were projected for ten years out if effective interventions and preventive treatments for the condition are not identified and widely available.

Their forecasts for ASD-related medical, nonmedical and productivity losses are $268 billion for 2015 and $461 billion for 2025. The researchers noted that these estimates are conservative and, if ASD prevalence continues to increase as it has in recent years, the costs could reach $1 trillion by 2025.[275]

Looking for justice? The US Department of Justice has jurisdiction, but it has been recruited to defend HHS against any vaccine injury claim, even though the vaccine injury compensation program was intended to be no-fault. Over the years, HHS has systematically eliminated any vaccine-injury category for which a child could seek compensation. It is now virtually impossible for a child to receive compensation for a vaccine injury. Every time HHS paid out a claim, the condition that allowed that injured child to tap into the compensation program was eliminated as being a compensatory condition for subsequent claimants. It is an ironic reality that we now live in a country where the dissemination of a known poison and the disinformation surrounding it is being used against us as if we were the enemies in some military campaign.

We have become enemy combatants. This goes beyond just individuals who do not want to lose their jobs or accept culpability that might injure their careers. Removing thimerosal from vaccines does not destroy the vaccination program, but it does require the infrastructure to change, and there are organizations that simply do not want that change to take place, so they made sure it is being added back into the vaccine schedule in the form of the flu vaccine. Disinformation surrounding this issue is as much a danger as the mercury, but where there is danger, there is also opportunity. However, the public can perceive only what is shown to them. More galling than anything has been the effort to keep the public from knowing, and the intimidation of many to violate the public trust.

Regrettably, it seems that we have entrusted the public safety to others whose conscious awareness of the common well-being often fades in the face of compromising interests. Illogically, these individuals have put these interests above children and grandchildren—except for those like Dr. Johnston, who was clear about protecting his own family. Dick Johnston, MD, University of Colorado School of Medicine and National Jewish Center was chairman of the Simpsonwood meeting that met in June of 2000 to review Verstraeten's Phase One/Generation Zero data. This is what he said at the meeting (p. 198):

Forgive this personal comment, but I got called out at eight o'clock for an emergency call and my daughter-in-law delivered a son by C-section. Our first male in the line of the next generation, and I do not want that grandson to get a Thimerosal-containing vaccine until we know better what is going on. It will probably take a long time. In the meantime, and I know there are probably implications for this internationally, but in the meantime I think I want that grandson to only be given Thimerosal-free vaccines.

In 2008, I resigned from the American Academy of Pediatrics, where I had been a fellow for two decades.

This is what I wrote:

As a pediatrician, who has been a fellow of the American Academy of Pediatrics (AAP) for two decades, I find the AAP's approach to the autism epidemic to be deeply disturbing. Not only have they allowed the myth of better diagnosing (as the reason for all the notice given to affected children) to be perpetuated, but when they were put on notice at the Centers for Disease Control and Prevention's (CDC's) Simpsonwood meeting in 2000, that the mercury in the preservative Thimerosal was causing speech delays and learning disabilities, they obfuscated and hid that information. They never made good on their 1999 pledge to have Thimerosal eliminated from vaccines and almost a decade later joined in the protest against a fictitious TV show (Eli Stone) because it was critical of mercury being in vaccines.

Out of about 120 million doses of the worthless[276] flu vaccine shipped for the 2007–08 flu season, no more than about 15 million doses, including the less than 4 million live-virus doses, were no-Thimerosal doses.

That means that about 87% contained some level of Thimerosal and at least 42% contained the maximum level (0.01%) of Thimerosal. If a pregnant woman got a flu shot in 2001 and her child followed the flu shot recommendations, the baby/fetus would have received six flu shots with the full amount of Thimerosal by the year 2005.

Today, in some states, the flu vaccine given to those under 3 years of age is supposed to contain no more than a trace level of Thimerosal, but with no government agency testing vaccines for mercury, the only ones who know whether a preservative free vaccine (flu or otherwise) is actually mercury-free are the manufacturers themselves.

Vaccines with "trace" amounts of Thimerosal, by definition, "contain less than 1 microgram of mercury (Hg) per dose."[277] For example, consider that the reduced-Thimerosal flu vaccine with 0.0002% mercury is equivalent to 1 microgram (μg) of Hg per 0.5 mL, or 2 μg of Hg per mL, which is the same as 2000 μg per liter; or 2000 ppb or parts per billion.[278]

0.5 parts per billion (ppb) mercury has been shown to kill human neuroblastoma cells.[279]

2 ppb mercury is the U.S. EPA limit for drinking water.[280]

20 ppb mercury destroys neurite membrane structures.[281]

200 ppb mercury is the level in liquid that the EPA classifies as hazardous waste.[282]

25,000 ppb mercury is the concentration of mercury in multi-dose, hepatitis B vaccine vials, administered at birth from 1991–2001 in the U.S.

50,000 ppb mercury is the concentration of mercury in multi-dose DTP and haemophilus B vaccine vials, administered 8 times in the 1990's to children at 2, 4, 6, 12, and 18 months of age and currently "preservative" level mercury in multi-dose flu, meningococcal, and tetanus (7 and older) vaccines.

For years the Infectious Disease division at the CDC (and others) has said the reason for the dramatic increase in autism is due to "better diagnosing" and "greater awareness." They have encouraged those like the AAP to manufacture uncertainty by publishing articles that were less than truthful. The AAP shamefully played along, perhaps encouraged by the largesse of vaccine manufacturers who significantly contribute to the AAP's yearly budget. To publish studies that showed the removal of a known neurotoxin (mercury) from vaccine-caused the incidence of autism to increase was shameful pseudo-science.

There is another budget to consider for 80 percent of autistic Americans under the age of 18, and we will soon begin to see a dramatic impact on Social Security in coming years as these children become dependent adults. There are no studies that have found the previously undiagnosed or misdiagnosed autistic individuals among older Americans. They simply aren't there. So what is coming will significantly impact society. Since there are no genetic epidemics, this leaves an epidemic linked to some sort of exposure. Now, the increase of autism has been linked to the increase in mercury exposure through fish and industrial sources, amalgam and additionally, through increased parenteral exposure to Thimerosal—no controlled, randomized study regarding the safety of amalgam or Thimerosal exists.

A Scientific Consensus Statement on Environmental Agents Associated with Neurodevelopmental Disorders (by the Collaborative on Health and the Environment's Learning and Developmental Disabilities Initiative) concludes that environmental contaminants are an important cause of learning and developmental disabilities. Delayed detoxification of mercury severely impairs methylation reactions (required for the correct expression of DNA, RNA, and neurotransmitters), which further adversely affects growth factor derived development of the brain and attention abilities. Phospholipid methylation, which is crucial for attention, is impaired in autistic and attention deficit hyperactivity disorders.

In a first analysis of the VSD datasets,[283] Verstraeten had described a 7.6 to 11.4 fold increase of autism risk in children at one month, with the highest mercury exposure levels compared to children with no exposure. In four subsequent separate generations of the analysis, which involve the exclusion of children with no Thimerosal exposure and less than two polio vaccines, the statistical significance disappeared. This is what was published by the AAP even though they knew the truth. How did they know the truth?

Again, the data were presented at the Simpsonwood meeting in June 2000, a meeting that was illegal to hold. No Federal agency is allowed to call a meeting together with representatives of private industry (all the vaccine manufacturers were represented at this meeting) without opening the meeting to the public. Thimerosal was tested only once, by Eli Lilly on 22 adult patients suffering from meningitis. There was no chance for follow-up to observe long-term effects, as all of the patients in this "study" died. Even if follow-up had been possible, damage to the developing brains of very young children would have remained an unknown. Eli Lilly said it was safe and the medical community accepted it.

After the creation of the FDA, its use was simply continued. The federal government has never tested the type of mercury in vaccines for toxicity. This is an unconscionable oversight failure at best, at worse it is an example of how we have left consensus reality to be created by the liars, thieves, cheats, killers, and the junk scientists they employ. How it came to pass that the AAP joined these rogues and became an active participant in this skullduggery is beyond reason—even beyond greed. They have remained silent as mercury-laden vaccine continues to be exported and used in all third world and second world countries.

We are living in a time where an incredible overplay of lies, self-aggrandizing behavior and non-science are the norm. We have tolerated the junk science that has covered up the true cause of this epidemic at a considerable cost to science, the public, and our very way of life in this country. Is it a stretch to suggest that by putting our collective heads in the sand about the autism epidemic we have made it possible for the COVIDians to destroy our very civilization?

Then ask why haven't pediatricians come forward to demand the end of the use of Thimerosal once and for all, and to advocate for the treatment of these children before it is too late? Why are they not at the front of the line protesting the amounts of mercury allowed to come out of coal-fired power plants?

Why aren't they leading the charge to stop the use of mercury amalgam dental fillings that are placed in the mouths of young children and pregnant women?

The very Federal agencies that should have been sounding the alarm bell about environmental pollution creating future generations of mentally disabled citizens did less than remain silent because they have become arms of the very corporations that profit from selling and distributing poisons. Just look who sits on the FDA's Scientific Advisory Boards—the conflicts of interest are so glaring as to suggest that the FDA has become a trade arm of Big Pharma.

I will no longer enable the AAP to be party to the damage that is being done to the world's children by sending in my dues for a third decade. It is a token protest, but it has to begin with someone.

# 7

# The Religion of Jabism: A Special Chapter on Vaccines

*"FDA is inherently biased in favor of the pharmaceutical industry. It views industry as its client, whose interests it must represent and advance. It views its primary mission as approving as many drugs it can, regardless of whether the drugs are safe or needed."*[284]

— David J. Graham, American epidemiologist, Associate Director of the Food and Drug Administration's (FDA) Office of Drug Safety

The Bill and Melinda Gates Foundation is the perfect model of effective altruism. Mr. Gates was recorded saying vaccines will help reduce the world's population by 10 percent (via sterilization campaigns secretly implemented using vaccines). "If we do a really great job on new vaccines . . . we could lower [world population] by 10 or 15 percent."[285] Gates has often bragged about how he gets a 20:1 return on his foundation's investments on vaccines.

It would also be commendable if those who promote vaccine actually knew what they were doing, but they don't. Name one recent randomized clinical trial documenting the effect on child mortality of any of the existing vaccines or combination of vaccines (because no child gets just one vaccine; they get many, and often at once) that showed a decrease in mortality. There is no study so it can't be named.

I can name a randomized clinical vaccine trial that resulted in a 33 percent increase in mortality among children aged four to sixty months in using the high-titer MMR with the DTaP (the Aaby et al. study).[286] The good old United States, the most-vaccinated nation on the planet, has the worst infant mortality of any First World nation.[287]

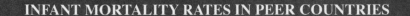

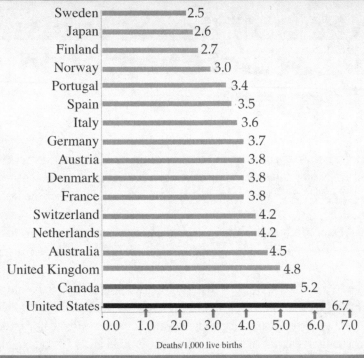

## INFANT MORTALITY RATES IN PEER COUNTRIES

| Country | Rate |
|---|---|
| Sweden | 2.5 |
| Japan | 2.6 |
| Finland | 2.7 |
| Norway | 3.0 |
| Portugal | 3.4 |
| Spain | 3.5 |
| Italy | 3.6 |
| Germany | 3.7 |
| Austria | 3.8 |
| Denmark | 3.8 |
| France | 3.8 |
| Switzerland | 4.2 |
| Netherlands | 4.2 |
| Australia | 4.5 |
| United Kingdom | 4.8 |
| Canada | 5.2 |
| United States | 6.7 |

Deaths/1,000 live births

NOTE: Rates averaged over 2005-2009    SOURCE: Data from OECD (2012c).

Infant mortality rates in 17 peer countries, 2005–2009. From the article "Graph of the Day: The United States Has a Really High Infant Mortality Rate" by Sarah Kliff, *Washington Post*, January 9, 2013 (http://www.washingtonpost.com/blogs/wonkblog/wp/2013/01/09/graph-of-the-day-the-united-states-has-a-really-high-infant-mortality-rate)

If a vaccine is shown to produce antibodies against a specific component of a virus or bacteria, it is considered to be effective, even if it neither prevents transmission of the disease nor infection. With COVID none of the jabs were even evaluated to see if they would prevent infection or transmission. Authorities use estimates and guesstimates about how many lives they will be saving using the vaccine based on its ability to create antibodies.[288] At best the purpose of vaccines is to make money, no need to find out if they cause harm or even work.

I believe vaccines have their place in the medical armamentarium—a small place that needs to be precise and controlled. But today we have the one-size-fits-all shotgun approach, the damn-the-torpedoes approach (on the way to the bank) encouraged by eugenics. If you go back seventy years to the 1940s and 1950s, there were six controlled trials including 45,662 children in the United States and the United Kingdom in which the BCG vaccine (not used in the United States) reduced mortality from causes other than tuberculosis by 25 percent (6 percent to 41 percent).[289] This was a good thing.

I have always felt the original intention of vaccines was a good one, but that has changed over the years, and making and selling vaccines has become a very big business where there is no liability and the only incentive is to sell more and more often.

We have the wrong people making vaccines, the wrong people testing vaccines, and the wrong people recommending vaccines—it just doesn't get any worse. No one is studying the effect of vaccines on overall morbidity and mortality in real-life situations, because if they did, they would find that vaccines, as they have been administered, have a direct link to neurodevelopmental syndromes (including autism) and now cause far more problems than they solve.

What was once a well-intentioned intervention ceased to provide any potential benefit, in part because there has been no consideration given to all the synergistic interactions these vaccines evoke (the biosemiotics of vaccines): the lack of knowledge of metal toxicology, sex difference, age differences, or ethnic differences. For example, the Aaby et al. study showed that when the timing of measles vaccine changed and DTP was administered after high-titer measles vaccine, female mortality increased. We have given a gun to a four-year-old in a sense. "They" don't have any financial incentive to really find out what they are doing because it has been decided that the public better not find out what was done and continues to be done by the mass use of vaccines.

While I don't like making sweeping generalizations, vaccines are such a scourge on our health that little more needs to be said about them because the mainstream (conventional) medical community—which knows next to nothing about vaccines—is so utterly brainwashed about vaccines that there is no way to reach them. "The science is in" they will say; "vaccines are safe" they will say; "vaccines are the greatest medical intervention in the last millennium and save so many lives" they will say. They believe this with such a passion that it makes you wonder where it comes from. The contents of vaccines, how they work, and how they are tested is actually a complete mystery to most physicians; they are clueless but for the programmed mantras they are trained to repeat.

So, how do vaccines work? Or don't work?

## POLIO

IPV (inactivated poliovirus vaccine)—the polio vaccine given in the United States cannot prevent transmission of poliovirus. Wild poliovirus eradication is attributed to the use of a different vaccine, OPV, or oral poliovirus vaccine. The IPV is given because it prevents polio infection from progressing to viremia (a generalized full-body viral infection because the virus got into the bloodstream) and thus protects motor neurons, removing the risk of bulbar polio and postpolio syndromes. OPV is not used in the United States because there is a risk it will convert back to wild polio under certain conditions. As previously revealed, pesticides are the real problem, along with a host on nonpolio EVs, but this section is about how vaccines work (or don't work).

## TETANUS

*C. tetani* spores can infect deep puncture wounds, but vaccinating for tetanus (via the DTaP combination vaccine) is about personal protection only. If you get a wound that is high risk for tetanus, and if you go to an emergency room, urgent care, or any other medical facility, you will be told you need a tetanus vaccine. But it will take a good two weeks for that vaccine to start generating protective antibodies—worthless for your current wound: you need tetanus immunoglobin, not the vaccine, if you think there is a high-risk wound. How many healthcare workers know that?

## DIPHTHERIA

The diphtheria toxoid vaccine (also contained in the DTaP vaccine) does not prevent or transmission of *C. diphtheriae*. Vaccinating for diphtheria helps one's body neutralize the toxin created by the bacteria. That is all it does: you personally won't get as sick, because this is a personal health intervention. It does not stop you from getting infected or infecting someone else.

## PERTUSSIS

The acellular pertussis (aP) vaccine (the last piece of the combo DTaP vaccine) is not capable of preventing infection or transmission of *B. pertussis,* and even the FDA has issued a warning about this. But pertussis variants (PRN-negative strains) currently in circulation are at an advantage for infecting vaccinated children. In other words, the fully vaccinated are more likely to be infected, and thus contagious, than people who are not vaccinated.

In a 2015, a study in *BMC Medicine* authored by Benjamin M. Althouse and Samuel V. Scarpino used whooping cough case counts from the CDC, genomic data on the pertussis bacteria, and a detailed epidemiological model of whooping cough transmission to conclude that acellular vaccines may well have contributed to and been exacerbated by pertussis outbreaks by allowing infected individuals without symptoms to unknowingly spread pertussis multiple times.[290]

Their results also suggest that a practice called cocooning, where mothers, fathers, and siblings are vaccinated to protect newborns, isn't effective. "It just doesn't work, because even if you get the acellular vaccine you can still become infected and can still transmit. So that baby is not protected," Althouse said.

We now have a situation where it is imperative to vaccinate our children with this vaccine to protect them from the vaccinated, because it is the vaccinated that spread the disease. The current vaccine turns the newly vaccinated into pertussis factories for weeks or more at a time every time the child is vaccinated.

While it is true getting the vaccine protects the vaccinated from getting sick or as sick as they could get if they were unvaccinated, it is the vaccine that is now causing the spread of the illness. This in turn causes public health authorities to want to recommend vaccinating more and more often, when what they should be doing is creating a better vaccine.

## HAEMOPHILUS INFLUENZAE

The *H. influenzae* (a bacterium, not a virus) or Hib vaccine covers only the type b strain. This vaccine actually seemed to work and do its job well, because when I was a resident in pediatrics treating *H. influenzae,* meningitis was an almost daily event. The vaccine came out, and poof, we never saw another case. Of all the vaccines that are given to children, this is the one I was the most impressed with.

Yet over time, strain dominance shifted toward other types of *H. influenzae* (types a through f). This actually placed the general population, especially adults, more at risk for this infection than prior to giving the Hib to infants, and that is a public health trade-off some would make. Still, now that we know about the trade-off, these matters should be discussed openly, and it certainly doesn't make sense to blame non-vaccinated children for non–type b Hib infections.

## HEPATITIS B

Vaccinating infants for hepatitis B is about money, not public health. Infants are not at risk for getting hep B unless their mother has chronic untreated hep B (about two hundred cases a year in the United States), but if she didn't, there is no good reason to give this vaccine to an infant or a child. The chance is that twenty years later, should that child have a high-risk lifestyle, such as being a paramedic who gets exposed to a lot of blood, hep B vaccine given as an infant really won't be working anymore.

Among children who respond to the complete primary 3-dose vaccination series with anti-HBs concentrations of >10 mIU/mL, 15% to 50% have low or undetectable concentrations of anti-HBs 5–15 years after the start of the vaccination series.

In adults, anti-HBs concentrations decrease rapidly within the first year after primary vaccination and more slowly thereafter. A decrease was noticed to a level of <10 mIU/mL in 7% to 50% of vaccinated adults within five years after vaccination and in 30% to 60% within 9–11 years after vaccination.[291]

In other words, this vaccine does not work in the population it is mandated to be given to—children—because it wears off so fast. If healthcare workers are required to get it, they probably should be getting it every five years.

## MMR

No need to explain how a vaccine works when it doesn't (mumps). Some components of the MMR have been shown to have no efficacy, and this is now the subject of an ongoing False Claims Act violation against Merck by two former virologists, Stephen Krahling and Joan Wlochowski. They claim that Merck markets the MMR vaccines under false pretenses. Apparently, the MMR is mislabeled, misbranded, adulterated, and falsely certified as having a 95 percent efficacy rate.

Merck allegedly manipulated test results for decades in order to create a false 95 percent efficacy rate for the mumps component of their multivalent MMR vaccines.

The former Merck virologists contend that the multivalent MMR has a vastly reduced efficacy that is directly responsible for mumps outbreaks during the last decade, which prompted international calls for MMR booster shots every four to eight years.

But I can tell you how the MMR causes autism. The vaccine court has awarded compensation for this: Ryan Mojab, for example, suffered an injury under the Vaccine Injury Table (the list of illnesses compensable by the Vaccine Act), namely, an encephalitis within five to fifteen days following receipt of the MMR. Says the US Department of HHS regarding the case: "This case is appropriate for compensation." Ryan has autism as a result of his "encephalitis," but court records are sealed, so publicly all the government will admit to is that Ryan developed an encephalitis from the MMR. That is, they won't come out and say his encephalitis led to brain injury that gave him the symptoms the lay world calls autism. Why seal the records unless there is something there you don't want the public to know?

Oh, I love transparency! The government doesn't.

Look at what these two studies tell us:

- "Detection and Sequencing of Measles Virus from Peripheral Mononuclear Cells from Patients with Inflammatory Bowel Disease and Autism" *Digestive Diseases and Sciences*, 2000, Hisashi Kawashima, Takayuki Mori, Yasuyo Kashiwagi, Kouji Takekuma.

This study shows that the measles in the bowels of autistic children is from the MMR vaccine.

> Additionally, a new syndrome has been reported in children with autism who exhibited developmental regression and gastrointestinal symptoms (autistic enterocolitis), in some cases soon after MMR vaccine. It is not known whether the virus, if confirmed to be present in these patients, derives from either wild strains or vaccine strains. . . . The sequences obtained from the patients with ulcerative colitis and children with autism were consistent with being vaccine strains. The results were concordant with the exposure history of the patients. Persistence of measles virus was confirmed in PBMC in some patients with chronic intestinal inflammation.

- "Dysregulated Innate Immune Responses in Young Children with Autism Spectrum Disorders: Their Relationship to Gastrointestinal Symptoms and Dietary Intervention" *Neuropsychobiology*, 2005, Harumi Jyonouchi, MD (New Jersey Medical School). This study examines the link between autistic behaviors and gastrointestinal disorders and notes a possible link "between GI and behavioral symptoms mediated by innate immune abnormalities."

Notice that Dr. Andrew Wakefield didn't have anything to do with the above research papers. Wakefield has been inappropriately turned into a scapegoat for the highly controversial study published in the medical journal the *Lancet* in 1998. Dr. Wakefield worked with Professor John Walker-Smith, who received funding to appeal the GMC (General Medical Council) decision from his insurance carrier, while Dr. Wakefield did not—and was therefore unable to mount an appeal in the high court. His research was not fraudulent, and his co-author has already been exonerated. Judge John Mitting's conclusion, from an appeal by the highly respected pediatric gastroenterologist Professor John Walker-Smith, stated, "Both on general issues and the *Lancet* paper and in relation to individual children, the panel's overall conclusion that Professor Walker-Smith was guilty of serious professional misconduct was flawed. . . . The panel's determination cannot stand. I therefore quash it."

Religions can't stand up to transparency. Anyone, be they a physician (Andrew Wakefield) or a lawyer (RFK Jr.) who dares question the religion of Jabism[292] is personally attacked. Remember, the Magisterium of Jabism employs a horde of running humans to counter, discredit, and disembowel anyone who crosses them.

In the context of a religion, you can believe whatever you want.

So, despite what vaccinists and their religion of Jabism believe, what if the Magisterium of Jabism—the CDC, vaccine manufacturers, and their high priests, such as Dr. Paul Profit—know how dangerous vaccines are, and they do, yet purposely discounted these dangers publicly because of greed or some other even more sinful agenda, such as population control, then aren't they criminals?

With the assistance of the controlled lame-stream media, the unsound mythoi of Jabism continues to be praised and proselytized because major media channels are bought and paid for by the same transnational corporations that give the orders for just about everything important.

The heretic whistle-blower Dr. William Thompson (previously mentioned in chapter 6) released thousands of pages of CDC documents with research data that unveiled the agency's long history of falsified studies and that concealed the serious miscarriages of science, all in the name of the unholy vaccine.

Dr. Thompson confessed he was part of the CDC's treachery to obscure evidence proving that thimerosal, as well as the MMR vaccine, are directly linked to autism.

You haven't heard about Dr. Thompson?

Is that a surprise when 70 percent of the media's ad revenue is paid by pharmaceutical companies in nonelection years? What do they do with a chap like Thompson? Too many people know about him for him to turn up wet in some bushes, but maybe a plane crash will be called up. Just make sure no one in Congress ever calls for a hearing.

John Rappoport's blog gives a few reasons why those who manipulate the Jabists want to force everyone to be vaccinated. I found seven of his reasons compelling:

One: Secure compliance from citizens. Induce them to obey orders.

Two: Because vaccines are unavoidably unsafe (as per the Supreme Court), obedience becomes debilitation—you can't rise up to fight tyranny when you are sick.

Three: In the "developing world," where megacorporations plunder cheap labor and mineral resources, vaccines become subterfuge for the real problems:

enforced poverty, provoked war, chronically contaminated water supplies, lack of basic sanitation, stolen land, severe generation-to-generation malnutrition and starvation, overcrowding, and industrial pollution.

Four: Direct access (by needle) to every individual bloodstream in the world so that the depopulation vaccines can be given as they have been in the Philippines and Kenya—hormone (hCG) that causes miscarriages in women who later become pregnant. The altered vaccines are instruments of birth prevention and population control.

Five: The massive propaganda hailing the miraculous benefits of vaccination obscures very unpleasant truths about the crimes of the medical cartel. The strategy is simple: hog and clog the media with positive fairy tales about the medical cartel. Cover up the wholesale destruction. Vaccines must be seen by the public as the greatest medical breakthrough ever, where all vaccines are safe, all vaccines are effective, and all vaccines can be given to everyone, anytime and all the time.

Six: The money. Medical care and treatment is a multi-trillion-dollar business, globally.

Seven: Maintaining the all-important fiction that "disease is inevitably caused by germs and nothing else," the vaccine establishment can trumpet its fairy tale as the triumph of medical science in the war against germs. In doing so, it can, for example, divert attention from the toxic-illness effects of industrial pollution. Needless to say, this diversion is a major goal of polluting megacorporations who forward the goals of globalism.

## LOSING MY RELIGION

Every so often the modern religion of Jabism must create a reason to encourage the masses to submit to the almighty virus so that fear can be created and money can be made. Feed the machine! "Human sacrifice" may be a more apt term.

If in need of a reminder, there was that sacerdotal release of a lab-created virus in a poor suburb of Mexico City in 2009. How did a lab-created flu virus end up finding its way to a slummy part of Mexico City? Why was there no public outcry about a lab-created[293] H1N1 virus showing up in a slum in Mexico City? The CDC was too busy announcing how many people in the United States were going to die from this new flu. More fear to spread ahead of a new and profitable vaccine.

The WHO even changed their definition of a pandemic to make sure this new, man-made killer virus would get all the PR it needed, but the viral apocalypse never took place, and the declared pandemic never happened. It makes one wonder if the "conspiracy theories" that HIV found its way into the gay populations of NYC and San Francisco through the hep B vaccine trials in the late 1970s are more conspiracy facts (not theories).

HIV aside, it is so very interesting that Baxter Pharmaceutical was chosen by WHO to lead the efforts in finding a vaccine cure for H1N1. Baxter was responsible for sending flu vaccines contaminated with live H5N1 avian flu virus to eighteen countries and was injected into thousands of people before someone caught the mistake.

They wouldn't purposely want to create a pandemic, unless of course they already had the vaccine ready to go, making them the most logical company to produce the vaccine. It is just business after all.

The most fortunate coincidence was that Baxter had a manufacturing plant in Cuernavaca, just fifty miles from the H1N1 ground-zero outbreak in Mexico City.

The hallmark of any long-term organized conspiracy is compartmentalization. Each player is only aware of his small part.

Rising through the ranks, players see a bit more of the actual picture, but they continue to believe they are doing the right thing.

And there is always the threat of loss of status, money, job, future career (and even life and limb) to offset the desire to blow the whistle.

At upper levels, players understand still more of the whole picture. Few of them, however, are willing to grasp the intentionality of what is being visited on populations.

The top controllers are the contented psychopaths. They, too, believe they're doing the right thing—but their definition of "right" and "good" is unique. It involves widespread destruction.

Understanding all these points should convince those who resist vaccination that playing defense, hoping for acknowledgment, and pleading for understanding are not enough. Going on the offense with great energy is required.[294]

The cost of letting all this scientific malfeasance take place without accountability allowed the Great Democide of 2020 to go operational—so far, no one has been held accountable.

## INFLUENZA VACCINE

"No efficacy has been shown in young children (less than 2 years) or institutionalised elderly. . . . Safety data in children under years were absent."[295]

Depending upon which flu vaccine study you look at, the flu vaccine efficacy ranges from a low of 0 percent to a high of 20-something percent.

Every year the government spends $1 billion to purchase quasi-worthless, mercury-laden flu vaccine and then does its best to push it on everyone. In 2015, it was such a miss in terms of flu strains that the CDC had to admit it was basically a failure, but they wanted us to get it anyway because it was, after all, the best way to prevent the flu.

It is actually illegal for government officials to doublespeak (or at least it used to be), but when no one holds them accountable, do you think they care how often they say how nice the emperor's new clothes look? It is about money, yes; saving face, yes; but it is also about an agenda that can count on the public to roll up their sleeves whenever they say so and for whatever vaccine they scare us into taking.

In 2013 and 2014, vaccines accounted for over 93,000 adverse reactions, including 8,888 hospitalizations and 1,080 deaths, according to the government's Vaccine Adverse Events Reporting System (VAERS). Since VAERS accounts for only 10 percent of the actual adverse reactions,[296] that is a lot of collateral damage.

In Finland alone there were 800 cases of narcolepsy associated with Glaxo's flu vaccine Pandemrix. The FDA's response about mercury-laden flu vaccine being pushed on pregnant women was that it was not by their recommendation or approval but by the CDC's, and they left it at that.

I got the flu in 2015. I had just delivered a talk on Lyme disease at the biannual conference of the Medical Academy for Pediatric Special Needs. I went to bed feeling previral. I should have known something serious was going down because I couldn't stop watching a PBS special on Lawrence Welk. I didn't take my Alinia until the next morning when I was feeling more than just previral. Yes, Alinia has shown itself to be very efficacious against influenza, with Romark Pharmaceuticals already in Phase III clinical trials[297] (the last step required before the FDA would consider a new indication for Alinia).

The antiviral flu drugs consist of two classes of medications: adamantanes and neuraminidase inhibitors. In the United States, two adamantanes (amantadine and rimantidine) and two neuraminidase inhibitors (oseltamivir and zanamivir) are available. The antiviral ribavirin, which is approved for use against hepatitis C and RSV infections, also has activity against influenza.

With resistance to adamantanes now pervasive, the neuraminidase inhibitors are the primary treatment option; however, use of zanamivir is limited because it requires administration by an often cumbersome inhalation device. Of late, resistance to neuraminidase inhibitors has been limited, except during the 2008–09 seasonal influenza season, during which the seasonal H1N1 virus exhibited widespread resistance to oseltamivir. Thus, oseltamivir has the almost exclusive status as the antiviral of choice, even though it may be coming to the end of its usefulness because of resistance.

# A ROLE FOR ALINIA?

Alinia's ability to halt influenza viral replication is rather unusual and may not be subject to resistance. It needs to be started early to be most effective. Essentially you have to have it with you just as I did just for such an event. I went through a mini-flu—the flavor of all the flu stages in a mild form over a three-day period. But it was the flu, and had my immune system been in better shape, I probably would not have even had those symptoms. However, I was exhausted when I came down with the flu, and if not for the Alinia I would have been very sick.

No Alinia? There is still another way.

Epigallocatechin gallate (EGCG),[298] a catechin or polyphenol contained in green tea, has an inhibitory effect against all types of influenza viruses. It matters not whether it be the bird flu (H5N1), the Hong Kong flu, or that laboratory-created swine flu of 2009 (H1N1). It doesn't matter—it even suppressed viral RNA synthesis. The anti-influenza viral efficacy of EGCG is attributable to damage to the physical properties of the viral envelope and partial inhibition of the NA surface glycoprotein. The knowledge about this feature of green tea and its main active ingredient go back a quarter of a century in the medical literature. This is not new information, but it is new to most people because there is no pharmaceutical company making bank on EGCG, which cannot be patented.

Think about all the fearmongering that goes on each and every year by the CDC and others, such as all the major media newscasters, to get the public to inject themselves with the mercury-laden flu vaccine that one could argue (correctly) has questionable safety and marginal efficacy (that is giving the vaccine more credit than it is due) when there is something natural and benign. What is that about? Oh yeah, greed, etc.

EGCG can be taken to prevent the flu and treat the flu in its early stages. One may still need oil of oregano and garlic to minimize the bacterial respiratory infection that often comes with the flu for many, but the point is there has always been something nutritional to prevent and treat the flu. Once again we have been hornswoggled by a corrupt governmental agency acting as the running dogs of vaccine manufacturers who have taken them over. No one dies, no one gets sick, and no one is injured drinking green tea or taking EGCG extract.

Flu jabs or shots may be the biggest medical fraud of all time, but since the competition is so fierce for that position, I don't know if I can give it the official nod for being the biggest.

I would take close to two grams of EGCG every three to four hours if I thought I was coming down with the flu, and up to 50,000 IU of $D_3$ for a couple of days.

Clinical trials have found that vitamin D was extremely effective at halting influenza infections in children.[299] This was a double-blind, randomized controlled trial—the gold standard in medicine. It showed that vitamin D was 800 percent more effective than the flu vaccine at preventing influenza infections in children. An unexpected finding of the study was that vitamin D also reduced asthma in the children studied. The children received 1,200 IU (not 50,000 IU).

I hope by now no explanation is needed regarding why the CDC just isn't telling everyone to take extra vitamin $D_3$.

But wait, there is more!

Charles Hensley, the man who came up with spraying zinc in one's nose to prevent and treat the common cold, has a patent that is worth a read: Method and Composition for Preventing and Treating Avian Influenza in Poultry, United States Patent Application 20130253047.

A little alpha lipoic acid, a little EGCG, a little NAC, and then some theaflavin—only the best for the flock, eh? But what is this theaflavin?

Theaflavins are antioxidant polyphenols that are formed from the condensation of flavan-3-ols in tea leaves during the fermentation of black tea (EGCG will break down into some of the theaflavins in the liver): "Our results indicated that TF derivatives are potential compounds with anti-influenza viral replication and anti-inflammatory properties. These findings will provide important information for new drug design and development for the treatment of influenza virus infection."[300]

So, Alinia, EGCG, theaflavins, and resveratrol derivatives (according to some research) have anti-influenza properties. The point is there are some solid contenders for safe and efficacious flu prevention and treatment, and the flu vaccine isn't one of them.

If you are feeling abandoned by modern medicine—which not only keeps from the public important nutritional research that could treat and prevent various infections, but also constantly markets highly questionable products that have seriously lethal side effects—you are not alone. Nowhere is this more evident than in the effort to vaccinate the population against the HPV virus.

## THE HUMAN RIGHTS VIOLATION CALLED THE HPV VACCINE

I predict that Gardasil will become the greatest medical scandal of all times because at some point in time, the evidence will add up to prove that this vaccine, technical and scientific feat that it may be, has absolutely no effect on cervical cancer and that all the very many adverse effects which destroy lives and even kill, serve no other purpose than to generate profit for the manufacturer. . . . There is far too much financial interest for these medicines to be withdrawn.

Dr. Bernard Dalbergue, a former pharmaceutical industry physician with Garda-sil manufacturer Merck, said this in an interview published in the April 2014 issue of the French magazine *Principes de Santé*.

Cervical cancer, the second-most common cancer in young women, is particularly prone to be found in the downtrodden and in impoverished countries. But this is no endorsement for human papilloma virus (HPV) vaccines. In fact, this is about revealing that HPV vaccines were created for only one reason, and it wasn't as a humanitarian effort to minimize cervical cancer. It was created by greed to create income for both a pharmaceutical company and the US governmental agencies, the National Institutes of Health and Health and Human Services that owned the technology used in the vaccine under the cover of doing something beneficial—a "greater good." The HPV vaccine has less value than snake oil. At least snake oil is rich in omega-3 EFAs, and consuming snake oil won't harm anyone, but the same cannot be said for the HPV vaccine. The HPV vaccine was never necessary, and the true interventions available for those who are concerned about preventing cervical cancer have been suppressed.

## DOES HPV CAUSE CERVICAL CANCER?

While a virus may almost always be a trigger for cancer on a cellular/DNA level, it needs the environment, the internal milieu, to be prepared correctly to allow the wildcat cells to proliferate. Because the public doesn't know this, it is easy for trusted authorities to impose fear of the virus on the populace just as was done and is still done with the poliovirus. It is a tried and true method of disinformation. In the case of cervical cancer, the field upon which it takes hold must be deficient in certain vitamins. Without that deficiency, it is very unlikely cervical cancer will take hold. While it may remain controversial which vitamins, or combinations thereof, hold the key, the point is this is about a nutritional issue. But first let's look at some numbers:

- According to Merck's Gardasil 9 package insert, 3.3% of participants who were given Gardasil during the most recent clinical trials "experienced new medical conditions potentially indicative of autoimmune disorders." (recipients)
- According to a press release from Sanofi-Pasteur MSD dated June 17, 2015, 183 million doses of Gardasil have been distributed worldwide.
- Using Merck's own clinical trial percentage, this means there could be as many as 6,039,000 girls around the world suffering autoimmune conditions that could very well influence their health for the rest of their lives.

- According to the World Cancer Research Foundation, there were 528,000 cases of cervical cancer diagnosed worldwide (2012).

This is a vaccine that has never been proven to actually prevent even one case of cervical cancer, and yet we are willing to subject six million girls, based on the above, to an autoimmune disorder to potentially prevent half a million cases of cervical cancer?

Cervical cancer is a nutritional disorder that has a nutritional treatment, but such a treatment will not make a pharmaceutical company any money.

Indole-3-carbinol (I3C) is a phytochemical present in all members of the cruciferous vegetable family including cabbage, broccoli, brussels sprouts, cauliflower, and kale. In a double-blind, placebo-controlled study,[301] thirty patients with biopsy-confirmed cervical intraepithelial neoplasia (CIN), also known as cervical dysplasia, II-III, were randomized to receive placebo or 200 or 400 mg oral I3C daily for twelve weeks. None of the patients in the placebo group had complete regression of CIN. In contrast, four of eight patients in the 200-mg/day group and four of nine in the 400-mg/day group had complete regression of CIN based on twelve-week biopsy (400 mg/day is equivalent to one-third of a head of cabbage).

Adequate vitamin D levels need to be present as well, but the point is cervical cancer is far more about malnutrition than an HPV virus. The vitamin D connection is no surprise because adequate vitamin D levels are required to have the immune system deal with viral infections, and because most cancer patients are vitamin D deficient, regardless of what cancer they have, a vitamin D/cervical cancer connection is a foregone conclusion. Low vitamin D levels are not the only metabolic issue for cancer or pre-cancer patients, but it is a significant one.

Cigarette smoking, which is known to lower vitamin D levels, only adds to the risk of cervical cancer. The bottom line for women to understand is that an infection alone is an insufficient cause of cervical cancer. HPV is but only one risk factor along with cigarette smoking. There is no direct link between HPV and cervical cancer. The vast majority of women will get an HPV infection without getting cervical cancer, but in malnourished women, cervical cancer becomes a real risk. This is about poverty and nutrition—that is the direct link and the primary cause of cervical cancer.

## DO HPV VACCINES BENEFIT WOMEN'S HEALTH?

Those who care about a woman's risk of cervical cancer would do better to empower women everywhere and provide adequate nourishment, but this isn't about caring about or for women—this is just about profit. There has always been a pharmaceutical treatment for HPV infections (except in the United States).[302] One study showed that with just a ten-day course of therapy with this extremely benign drug (inosine pranobex, or Isoprinosine), there was an almost 80 percent elimination of HPV 16 and 18 in cervical cancer (CIN I-III) and pre-invasive cancer of the cervix and of those with recurrent CIN or Ca in situ in the remaining part of the cervix who were infected with HPV.[303] This study was published the same year the FDA fast tracked the HPV vaccine.

The vaccines cover HPV 16 and 18, responsible for being the trigger for 70 percent of cervical cancers, but no one actually knows if the vaccine prevents infection (let alone cancer). All we know is they increase antibodies to those two viral strains for an unspecified period of time. The vaccines do not cover sixteen other HPV strains that can trigger genital cancer (31, 45, 33, 35, 39, 51, 52, 56, 58, 59, 26, 53, 66, 68, 73, 82).[304] We do know getting the vaccine actually increases the risk of getting carcinoma in situ lesions from HPV strains not covered by the vaccine.[305]

Now this bears repeating: the FDA apparently knew the vaccine actually increased cervical cancer risk by 40 percent in women who had already been exposed to HPV and used magical thinking (no scientific evidence) to deal with this problem by recommending approving the vaccine for young girls hoping (I can only assume) they were never exposed. But the evidence is that infants can be exposed during the birth process, and since no testing of HPV serology is done before an HPV vaccine is given, nor is it required, the FDA's decision was irrational until you understand they were doing the bidding of not just Merck but the Health and Human Services Department that owns patents connected to this vaccine and would benefit if the vaccine became widely accepted.

In Japan[306] the evidence speaks for itself: Cervarix and Gardasil have been marketed in Japan since 2010. More than three million girls were inoculated with HPV vaccines until the cancelation of recommendation by Japanese Ministry of Health, Labor and Welfare (MHLW) in May 2013.

Incidence of serious adverse reactions to Cervarix, for example, was 3,300 cases per 100,000 person-years. Remember: there is no evidence yet that HPV vaccine decreases mortality from cervical cancer, but if for the sake of argument the HPV vaccine cuts the cervical cancer mortality by half, the expected maximum benefit would be 1.3 fewer deaths per 100,000 person-years.

The death rate of cervical cancer among white women is 2.1 per 100,000, 2.7 for Hispanic women, and 3.7 among black women, so if the vaccine was capable of cutting the mortality rate by 100 percent, it isn't even saving the life of three women per 100,000. Obviously, the harm (some of which is death) experienced is overwhelmingly greater than the expected maximum benefit of the vaccine.

This bears repeating: the vaccine will cause serious adverse reactions in 3,300 girls per 100,000 and prevent only two fewer deaths if the vaccine is assumed to prevent 100 percent of cancer cases in vaccinated individuals (and there is no evidence that it can save 1 percent of cancer cases from death).

While industry-sponsored studies will talk about antibody levels with no concern for safety, the Japan data brings home the true cost of this vaccine experiment and exercise in greed.

## ONE LESS BOY

Now that the HPV is recommended for boys, the deaths are starting. Joel Gomez, a fourteen-year-old healthy boy who had regular visits to the pediatrician's office for periodic checkups since birth, showed no evidence of any pre-existing health issues, specifically no evidence of cardiac abnormalities, psychological disorders, or substance abuse.

On June 19, 2013, Joel was given the first dose of Gardasil in his left arm in the doctor's office. No adverse reactions were reported following this first vaccination to either his family or his physician. On August 19, 2013, this boy was given a second injection of Gardasil as scheduled, and died in his sleep that night.

The autopsy report stated, "The Decedent died of myocarditis, which apparently was completely asymptomatic. By histology, the disease had been present for at least several days or weeks. The cause is unknown."[307]

So, what happened?

Sin Hang Lee, MD, Director Milford Molecular Diagnostics Laboratory and expert witness for the family, reviewed the microscopic slides and concluded that the lesion of the heart was a healing myocardial infarct of a few weeks old after the first Gardasil vaccination. In his opinion,[308]

> The HPV L1 gene DNA fragments bound to the aluminum adjuvant in Gardasil *can cause sudden and unexpected surge of tumor necrosis factor-α and other cytokines. Some of these cytokines released from macrophages are potent myocardial depressants, capable of causing hypotension with low cardiac perfusions in certain genetically or physically predisposed individuals.*

Cytokines are inflammatory molecules (little microscopic fire starters that come from while blood cells, called macrophages). Vaccinations can cause an immune response that is so out of control that it will cause a coagulation problem in the blood and the resultant clots cause strokes or in this case a heart attack. This out-of-control immune response can not only cause an increased clotting problem, but the antibodies can end up attacking parts of the body that resemble ingredients in the vaccine.

Imagine what a shower of little blood clots does to the brain of a young child.

Dr. Lee went on to write an open letter of complaint to Dr. Margret Chan, the director-general of the WHO, alleging misconduct and cover-up of HPV vaccine dangers by global health officials. The source of information for this was a trail of damning emails and other communication between global health officials obtained by Dr. Lee through a Freedom of Information Act (FOIA) request. The correspondence showed that global health officials knew that HPV vaccines Gardasil and Cervarix cause a dangerous inflammatory response greater than other vaccines but nevertheless reassured the public that the HPV vaccines were safe.

## MENINGITIS

Meningococcal group B meningitis is a rare illness that affects under 400 people per year nationally. The manufacturers' inserts predict that 1 percent to 1.3 percent of inoculated children will suffer "serious adverse effects." CDC's Epidemiology and Prevention of Vaccine-Preventable Diseases, also known as the Pink Book, forecasts that 0.3 percent of these will die from the vaccine. For every 100,000 school children that get this vaccine, 1,000 will become ill and three children will die in order to prevent around one person from contracting the disease. At between $84 and $117 per shot, and with the requirement for a two-shot series, the vaccine is a billion-dollar windfall for vaccine manufacturers often at taxpayer expense. In other words, in the name of helping children and young adults, the public is actually bankrolling what amounts to murder and sacrifice so vaccine manufactures that have no liability can make a lot of money.

Fact-check the above yourself, crunch the numbers, and then ponder what we have done, and ponder what we should be doing, and why we are not doing it.

## SCIENCE OR SUBTERFUGE?

Not only is the science behind this vaccine not present, but also the evidence shows cancer risk increased significantly. The fact that the NIH/DHHS-owned patents of the technology used in the vaccine, which was licensed to Merck, had everything to do with how this dangerous vaccine failed upward into approval and a fast track. This is a total loss of boundaries between corporation and state.

As of the present moment, the general public and the world need to understand that no scientific information coming from the NIH, CDC, FDA, or HHS can be trusted, nor policies created from them. The loss of confidence in these agencies is irrecoverable.

Any scientific publication that is authored by anyone coming from or funded by someone working for either the government or a pharmaceutical company can't be trusted.

Whether or not the subterfuge behind HPV vaccines constitutes a violation of human rights deserves its own discussion. Several states allow twelve-year-olds to receive this vaccine without parental consent. But a twelve-year-old cannot enter into a contract anywhere in the United States, so how could she possibly give informed consent for a vaccine?

They can't—there is no longer informed consent. We let that right be taken away. Remember: Liberty is not something one is given; liberty is only something someone takes from you. One does not give away the right to say no to vaccines that aren't even on the market yet. If you give away the right to informed consent, then that spills over into other areas you never intended it to spill over into.

Again, this aspect of the problem deserves international attention if not international legal intervention, but that is not taking place yet.

Which brings us to an even more troubling subject: the secretary of the Department of HHS can now declare a pandemic emergency for which a vaccine is a "countermeasure," thereby conferring liability protection on the vaccine manufacturer (or other countermeasure producer corporations).

In 2011, the Supreme Court in *Bruesewitz v. Wyeth* conferred much more sweeping immunity on the vaccine manufacturers based on the National Childhood Vaccine Injury Act/Program (NCVIP) without requiring an administration official to declare a pandemic emergency.

So, just as we are in a perpetual war against terrorism (except our own), we are in a permanent public health war—a de facto permanent public health emergency. We are turning into a public health police state in which all vaccine mandates approved by the CDC are automatic. Exemptions are eliminated, and liability for injury doesn't exist because vaccines are "countermeasures."[309]

We are the enemy, we must show our (vaccine) papers, and we must show no resistance—or else.

But what is driving this besides money? Greed is such an obvious answer that one often stops there. Another answer is the depopulation agenda of the UN and WHO, demonstrated by putting hCG into the vaccines to functionally sterilize women in many countries. But what if there was something even worse than that?

## WHERE IS THIS GOING?

It is time to call a spade a shovel and put on the table that offensive biological warfare research has never stopped in the United States. It is not just of historic interest. It is not illegal to have biodefense research programs—that is, vaccines. Under the cover of vaccines, the vaccine program, and biodefense programs, an illegal biological warfare program has been under way, which would completely explain both the irrational interest in pushing vaccines and why no one is to say one critical word about vaccines. This is all about biological warfare research and stockpiling of agents that are in violation of the BWC treaty signed off by Nixon in 1972. There were forty-six biolabs in Ukraine being operated by the US DOD, which is only interested in weapons and not public health, unless public health can be weaponized.

This topic is beyond the scope of this book, but could it be possible that part of the interest in ensuring everyone is vaccinated—often and for everything and anything that a vaccine comes on the market, such as—CoV2 to use a current example—not only will people blindly take the COVID vaccine without even asking if it prevents transmission or infection, but may be unaware their immune systems will be primed for an adverse event from the new jab.

Using one's imagination, what might happen if Ebola or Marburg breaks out big-time and the government orders every man, woman, and child to be vaccinated with a special Marburg or Ebola vaccine—no questions asked or else one gets shipped off to a FEMA camp, never to be seen again (might as well be dramatic). Everyone gets this Ebola vaccine. Likely there will be lots of vaccine injuries from it, but too bad: national public health emergency, acceptable collateral damage. But wait. The vaccine contains a Trojan horse: something in the vaccine that will cause a fatal problem when it encounters the substance "they" release from the air. Implausible? Can you say 5 G? But 5 G is not all that necessary when the COVID jab had cancer virus SV40 sequences written into its modified mRNA. Can you say Turbo Cancer?

It doesn't have to be electromagnetic. "They" are spraying all the time and we don't stop them. We pretend they aren't doing it because "they" use names like "geoengineering" or SAI when what "they" mean is chemtrail spraying—something done with no regard to you and yours. We have been bypassed, because we are worthless bottom-feeders to "them," except for our tax dollars that pay for their black-ops programs by the trillions.[310]

Wouldn't you think such an expensive program, especially if it were controlled by the military, should be easy to find in their budget? Not if the money seems to go missing. Taxpayer money to the sum of $8.5 trillion—that's with a "T"—has been doled out by Congress to the Pentagon since 1996, money that has never been accounted for. Some will just call this fraud,[311] but it does cover a lot of black-op programs, secret underground bases, unconventional craft, biowarfare projects, and geoengineering, to name a few.

So, when we are willing to give away our rights to be vaccinated without exemption for vaccines that have negative efficacy, and for vaccines that don't even exist, what are we telling "them"?

In June 2015, an article appeared in the *Daily Mail:* "Tens of Thousands of Teenage Girls Believed to Have Fallen Ill with Debilitating Illnesses after Routine HPV Cervical Cancer Jab."[312] Of course, anyone in a position to investigate or regulate has already been compromised by pharmaceutical interests or was soon thereafter.

Over 90 percent of girls who complain about untoward symptoms after receiving the HPV vaccine will be told it is all in their head.

Denial is not a river in Egypt.

# 8

# On Diagnosing and Treating Toxic/ Infectious/Immune Encephalopathy and Other Chronic Illness

As was said in the introduction, the original intention for this book was to reveal a lot of vanguard interventions for the true causes of some of the maladies that afflict us. The conditions I focused on in this book share some similar if not overlapping causes or triggers. As I come to the end of *Incurable Us,* it seems that it would be helpful to provide the information on how to determine what these problems might be and provide a sample of some relevant interventions. In this chapter I want to lay out an overview of how one evaluates and treats someone with brain pathology (unrelated to acute trauma) or any chronic illness, be it environmentally triggered, vaccine-induced, infectious, or from some other immune-excitotoxicity issues.

What follows is a taste of what functional medicine is all about. This one chapter is hardly more than an introduction to this area. I have truncated the information so as not to repeat the interventions I have already discussed in some detail.

A functional-medicine physician doesn't just look to see what kind of bandage to put on a problem but attempts to uncover underlying causalities and treat them. For example, most psychiatrists are preoccupied with balancing neurotransmitters in the brain (using prescribing practices heavily guided by pharmaceutical companies). An integrative psychiatrist, on the other hand, would be interested in what is causing the imbalance in neurotransmitters as well. Why put a patient on an antidepressant if he has an illness (which one has to look for) for which the right antibiotics might very well resolve the depression? If a patient has a double MTFHR mutation, they need biologically active folic acid, not necessarily a drug that doesn't actually address the underlying metabolic issue. Yes, finding an integrative psychiatrist is a nontrivial matter—they don't grow on trees.

It is worth noting that the MTFHR genetic polymorphisms are associated with adverse events (bad reactions) to smallpox vaccination in two independent study samples, which is why the one-size-fits-all vaccine policy of the CDC is insanity and pseudoscience.[313] Forced vaccinations are criminal, but that's where we could be heading, making the eugenics lobby exceedingly gleeful, because this is about population control, and not just money, as has already been described.

Be that as it may, you won't be able to go to your closest "doc-in-a-box" and expect them to understand this workup, nor will your HMO physician who has been allotted seven to ten minutes to see you be the person to help you with this. Furthermore, some of these tests require special kits from the labs, which have to be ordered in advance. Many naturopaths, chiropractors, and doctors of oriental medicine may be a better "go-to" person to help you with this process than your MD or DO types.

This information is here to help you know the kinds of tests that are relevant to a functional-medicine physician in evaluating and treating in this area. Knowledge is power.

## DIAGNOSTICS

### Biomarkers

Below is a list of lab testing that could be done, not for academic reasons, but to fine-tune potential interventions. There may be some overlap between certain panels, and I am not suggesting that everyone get all the tests at once, but this is a guide into what a functional-medicine workup should look like. It may look like a lot of testing, but I am sure there will be those who will be critical that I didn't list more.

### Genetic Testing

At the current moment, the most practical and affordable form of genetic testing is to look at single nucleotide polymorphisms (SNPs)—mutations in our genes that may make us more or less able to deal with the world we live in. We have genes that deal with detoxification, clotting, the immune system, and nutritional issues. It would be nice if Dr. McCoy from *Star Trek* could just zap us all with some futuristic device, but we are not there yet, and we have to go through the trouble of doing the testing, like peeling the layer of an onion and dealing with whatever is under that layer step by step.

The 23&Me test (which reports on your ancestral genetics: https://www.23andme.com) looks at millions of SNPs for under $200, and while most of the SNPs mean nothing or we don't know their relevance, it could be important information to have. Third-party applications help organize the genes in groups, such as the variance reports generated by livewello.com using the 23&Me raw data. With the assistance of someone knowledgeable in this area, such as someone with whom you can discuss the methylation cycle if you have a double MTFHR mutation, then you will be ahead of the game. The LiveWello folks have just such an application.

Below are the types of results you can receive from a DNA test.

- **Detoxification genomics** identifies genetic predispositions to altered detoxification. Common impairments include methylation, glutathione conjugation, acetylation, apolipoprotein E, and various cytochromes. Genova Diagnostics (Metametrix) has a detoxification profile,[314] but all these SNPs are also revealed in the raw data from 23&Me as well. For example, if over half the children with "autism" have poor levels of glutathione, then it is only logical to supplement this important peptide, especially if there is a mutation on the glutathione S-transferase gene.

    It is that simple: Identify a genetic weakness and compensate for any potential problem nutritionally. There is no guarantee that it will solve all of your problems or even any of your problems. But if you are trying to detox from poisons, then you want more glutathione, not less, and it is nice to have an objective reason for making the effort.

- **Lipid and clotting genomics** identifies genetic predispositions to altered blood-fat metabolism and clotting cascades. Altered lipid and clotting contributes to decreased blood flow to the tissues, especially the brain, resulting in impaired delivery of nutrients and oxygen to the affected areas. Genova Diagnostics (Metametrix) has their CV Health Profile and an interpretative guide: https://www.gdx.net/core/interpretive-guides/CVHealth-Genomic-Interp-Guide.pdf.

    Boston Heart Diagnostics has even more comprehensive panels to access overall risk of cardiovascular disease: http://www.bostonheartdiagnostics.com/hcp_better_risk.php).

    Genova has AssurePay, which caps the amount a patient might owe if her third-party payer bails on paying, and Boston Heart will hold only a (non-HMO) third-party payer responsible for remuneration.

**Immune genomics** looks at genes that modulate immune and inflammatory activity. These variations can affect balance between cell (Th-1) and humoral (Th-2) immunity. Common impairments include interleukin-1 beta, tissue necrosis factor alpha, and interleukins 4, 6, 10, and 13. Altered immune function contributes to increased inflammation, allergy, autoimmunity, and infection. For example, the gene that codes for IL-1ß (interleukin-1 beta) affects the duration and intensity of the acute inflammatory response. Having this knowledge may influence a practitioner to use one intervention over another to use for potential Herx reactions. For example, if you know that a patient is inclined to overproduce inflammatory cytokines, you prepare for that if you are treating Lyme.

## NUTRITIONAL BIOMARKERS AND TOXINS

Genova has their TRIAD panel that covers vitamin and mineral adequacy, insufficiencies in carnitine and NAC levels, oxidative stress and antioxidant sufficiency, detoxification adequacy, functional levels of B vitamins, neurotransmitter metabolism, mitochondrial energy production, lipoic acid and CoQ10 levels, specific markers of bacterial and yeast dysbiosis, essential amino acids sufficiency, food sensitivities, and intestinal hyperpermeability. A sample report can be found at www.gdx.net/core/sample-reports/TRIAD-SR.pdf.

Expect that 60 percent of autism spectrum children[315] will have at least one essential amino acid deficiency, and this group will most likely be deficient in valine, leucine, phenylalanine (produces tyrosine, dopamine, adrenal hormones), or lysine.

Great Plains Diagnostics (now called MosaicDx) came out with a very comprehensive organic toxin panel. It measures toxic exposure to pesticides and herbicides, as well as other fat-soluble toxins in the environment. Perhaps one of the most important tests to do first is a urine porphyrin profile. It directly reflects mitochondrial function and indirectly reflects environmental stressors such as heavy metals. Genova, Doctor's Data, and MosaicDx do this test. Porphyrin testing is used to identify abnormalities in hemoglobin synthesis. Classically, these abnormalities are associated with inherited errors of metabolism, but we now know environmental toxins can cause mitochondrial dysfunction, and it is in the mitochondria that porphyrins are made.

**Comprehensive cardiovascular assessment** evaluates blood fats, such as cholesterol and triglycerides, as well as inflammation and clot risk within the blood vessels. These markers can identify risk to the cardiovascular system but also may correlate with decreased circulation of blood to the smallest blood vessels in the brain. The so-called blood sludge theory states that highly viscous blood—caused by elevated blood fat and clotting factors—does not flow through the brain easily, causing a reduction of oxygen to the brain. Abnormalities are increasingly found in younger populations. Also, recent studies suggest that low cholesterol is involved in neurological disorders, including autism. The previously mentioned Boston Heart Panel is more than adequate for this area.

## INFECTIOUS DISEASE TESTING

- **Infection testing** measures both antibodies (immune proteins) against specific infectious organisms that are present *and* many viral levels (titers) directly. Chronic infections have been linked with numerous chronic diseases. It is theorized that these infections interfere with normal immune function and compromise cellular activity. Examples of organisms that are identified include *Mycoplasma pneumoniae, Chlamydia pneumoniae,* human herpes virus-6 (HHV-6), herpes simplex virus 1 and 2 (HSV 1 and 2), Epstein-Barr virus (EBV), *Borrelia burgdorferi* (Lyme disease), *Streptococcus, Aspergillus,* and rubella. All these titers can be obtained from conventional commercial labs, but not the Lyme test—only use IGeneX for Lyme testing (plus or minus ImmunoScience and DNA Connexions). InfectoLabs for looking at Lyme specific cytokines.
- **Streptococcal antibody panel** evaluates for the presence of streptococcal disease, including past infections of group A beta-hemolytic *Streptococcus*. In addition to classical manifestations—like rheumatic fever, scarlet fever, and kidney disease—high titers of these antibodies are associated with PANDAS (pediatric autoimmune neuropsychiatric disorder associated with streptococcal infections), autism spectrum disorders, and Tourette's syndrome.
- **The Mycoplasma Multiplex PCR Detection Kit** from www.clongen. com contains all the necessary ingredients for polymerase chain reaction for the amplification of a conserved region of the 16S ribosomal DNA of more than twenty-five different mycoplasma, acholeplasma, and ureaplasma.

  Fry Laboratories (http://frylabs.com) specializes in testing for and the identification of vector-borne and infectious organisms including (but not limited to) *Borreli, Bartonella, Ehrlichia, Anaplasma, Rickettsia, Babesia, Toxoplasma, Plasmodium* (malaria), *Trypanosoma,* infectious and/ or opportunistic protozoa, biofilm-forming pathogens, and newly emerging or recently recognized diseases. I use Fry when I suspect protozoal infections, as they can find them and their biofilm and provide the kind of documentation needed by many patients and their third-party payers.

## DIET

With the aim of minimizing inflammation in the body, an example diet would rely on eating organic vegetables, such as artichoke, asparagus, beets, bok choy, broccoli, cabbage, carrots, cauliflower, celery, chives, cucumbers, garlic, kale, kohlrabi, leeks, lettuce, mustard greens, onions, parsley, radishes, rhubarb, shallots, spinach, squash, sweet potatoes, water chestnuts, watercress, yams, and zucchini. Fermented vegetables, such as sauerkraut, are very good as long as they don't have added refined sugar or faux acidity from added vinegar. Fermented probiotic drinks are good as well.

What foods should be encouraged:

- **Meats:** organic beef—pasture or grass finished only, pasture raised (not just cage-free) chicken, fish (not farm raised and not from the Pacific), lamb, turkey. Swordfish, most tuna, and king mackerel are very high in mercury—avoid them almost completely. Select hormone-free and antibiotic-free chicken, turkey, and lamb.
- **Low glycemic organic fruits:** apples, apricots, avocados, berries, cherries, grapefruit, lemons, oranges, peaches, pears, and plums.
- **Herbs and spices:** organic basil, cilantro, coriander, garlic, ginger, mint, oregano, parsley, rosemary, sage, sea salt, and thyme. You will need to take an iodine supplement. Turmeric is one of the most important of all the spices.
- **Other:** apple cider vinegar, organic olive oil (the higher the biophenol count the better), olives, coconut oil, and water.

What foods to avoid:

- **Sugars:** including agave, candy, high fructose corn syrup, sucrose (also known as refined sugar or cane sugar). No aspartame in whatever name it is found, like AminoSweet.
- **Grains:** if you are not paleo and want grains in your diet, focus on the high grains such as millet and quinoa.
- **Nuts:** peanuts can have aflatoxins.
- **Gluten-containing foods:** even if you don't have an allergy to gluten, foods that contain gluten are bad for those with brain injuries or brain infections, and often are in foods that contain glyphosate.
- **Alcohol:** all alcohol should be avoided unless it is in a medicinal tincture.
- **Other:** canned foods, coffee, processed foods. Foods with high lectin counts such as raw kidney beans, raw soybeans, whole grains, and raw potatoes.

## SUPPLEMENTS

The following is a description of some of the most common supplements utilized and some explanation (many more could have been listed). They are not listed here to frustrate, because so much can be said about each one, but to provide a guide. This section is but an introduction into some of the tools used in functional medicine, especially as it relates to detoxification. There will always be someone who will have an untoward reaction to even the most benign herb, so if you have never taken something before, even if everyone else in the world is fine with it, take it initially at a low test dose and see how you do with it. That goes for antibiotics as well, unless you are in an emergency situation.

## AMINO ACIDS, MINERALS, AND PEPTIDES

- **Arginine** is an amino acid important for normal growth and development, energy storage, nitric oxide formation, and growth hormone production.
- **Carnitine** is an amino acid that primarily facilitates the process of beta-oxidation, which converts fat into energy. Carnitine deficiency is associated with mitochondrial dysfunction and impaired energy production.
- **Carnosine** is a dipeptide found in relatively high concentrations mainly in skeletal muscle, heart muscle, and nerve tissue, including the brain. Carnosine appears to have excellent antioxidant potential, produces nitric oxide, and may also act as a neurotransmitter.
- **Gama-aminobutyric acid (GABA)** is an inhibitory neurotransmitter in the brain and is used to balance excitatory responses, such as restlessness, irritability, insomnia, hyperactivity, and even seizures. GABA is able to induce relaxation, analgesia, and sleep.
- **Glutamine** is an amino acid used primarily for maintenance and repair of the small intestine. Since the small intestine is the site of nutrient absorption, glutamine is important in the treatment of malabsorption and leaky gut.
- **Glutathione (GSH)** is a powerful antioxidant and detoxifying agent. Although it is made in the body, genomic predispositions and environmental toxicity increase the requirement of this nutrient and necessitate its supplementation. It is the grease to our ball bearings. It won't fix those ball bearings, but if you have one that isn't working, you need more grease, not less.
- **5-Hydroxytryptophan (5-HTP)** is the activated form of tryptophan, which is an amino acid involved in the metabolism of serotonin and melatonin. It is used to support mood and sleep.

We are all on the spectrum of being poisoned to a greater or lesser degree. Those severely affected, if they are children, are often labeled as being on the autism spectrum. They are merely the canaries in the coal mine. We are all in the coal mine with them. Eighty percent of spectrum children lack up to 80 percent of normal levels of glutathione and its precursors, leaving none to spare for aggressive detoxification. For a successful recovery from heavy-metal-overload poisoning, the importance of additional glutathione and supplementation of essential fatty acids (fish oil, etc.) and antioxidants can't be overemphasized.

As with other cell types, the proliferation, growth, and differentiation of immune cells is dependent on GSH. The B-lymphocytes require adequate levels of intracellular GSH to differentiate, and healthy humans with relatively low lymphocyte GSH were found to have significantly lower CD4 counts. Intracellular GSH is also required for the T-cell proliferative response to mitogenic stimulation, for the activation of cytotoxic T "killer" cells, and for many specific T-cell functions, including DNA synthesis for cell replication as well as for the metabolism of interleukin-2, which is important for the mitogenic response. Experimental depletion of GSH inhibits immune cell functions, sometimes markedly, and in a number of different experimental systems the intracellular GSH of lymphocytes was shown to determine the magnitude of immunological capacity. These and other findings indicate that intracellular GSH status plays a central role in the functioning of immune cells. Interestingly, in those animals that could not make their own vitamin C (newborn rats, guinea pigs), GSH depletion was lethal. Supplementation of the diet with vitamin C protected these animals against GSH depletion and saved their lives.

GSH consumption from foods ranges from 25 to 125 milligrams per day. With the provision of sufficient amounts of sulfur, the liver will produce far more GSH (up to 14,000 milligrams per day) than what the diet provides. Sulfur-rich foods (garlic, eggs, asparagus, onions) may be lacking in various diets, and the provision of sulfur in food supplements (sulfur-bearing amino acids like N-acetyl cysteine, taurine, MSM, and lipoic acid) or GSH itself may be advantageous.

Liposomal or acetyl-L-GSH may be the most practical way to consume GSH. (One source to purchase from: http://naturedoc.com.)

- **Methylsulfonylmethane (MSM)** provides sulfur, a vital building block of joints, cartilage, skin, hair and nails, and methyl groups, which support many vital biochemical processes in the body, including energy production, neurochemistry metabolism, and detoxification. It is something that can be taken every day by almost everyone as if it were a vitamin. As with all high-sulfur compounds, they can promote yeast growth, so that has to be factored in.

- **N-acetyl cysteine (NAC)** is one of the most essential amino acids for detoxification. Containing a sulfur group, NAC is well-suited for assisting sulfation, which is a critical pathway for toxin elimination. NAC is also required for glutathione production within the body. But NAC can promote yeast growth.

- **S-adenosylmethionine (SAM-e)** is a primary methyl donor, involved in folic acid metabolism and brain chemistry. SAM-e is helpful as a supplement in those individuals with mood disorder and genomic polymorphisms (in the COMT gene) that are known to impair methylation.

- **Taurine** is an amino acid utilized by the liver for the production of bile, which is required for detoxification and fat absorption. Taurine is also a powerful water-soluble antioxidant.

## MINERALS

Minerals are critical components of cellular activity. Occurring both inside and outside of the cell, each mineral has specific functions within the body to promote healthy cellular activity.

- **Boron** assists with the activity of calcium within the body, including healthy bone formation. Boron may also improve mental functioning, strengthen the immune system, boost energy utilization, improve prostate health, and reduce cholesterol production.

- **Calcium** comes in many forms, which determines its absorbability (e.g., calcium citrate, malate, orotate, etc.). In addition to promoting bone health, calcium's electrical charge plays an important role in perpetuating the normal activity of many nerves. The movement of calcium ions (with its charge) through a nerve fiber (depolarization) constitutes the electrical wiring used to mediate a nerve impulse.

- **Chromium** is a trace mineral that helps the cell utilize blood glucose (sugar) and in this way assists in preventing or treating dysglycemia (blood sugar dysregulation), including diabetes.

- **Copper** is an important trace mineral involved in many physiologic activities, including the normal production of red blood cells. It is also used by cytosolic superoxide dismutase to scavenge free radicals within the body of the cell. Normal levels are important to avoid deficiency symptoms; however, high copper levels can be toxic. Copper therapy is closely monitored to avoid toxic levels.

- **Iron** is the central trace mineral in the formation of hemoglobin, which is the oxygen-carrying unit of red blood cells. Since iron is easily eliminated during detoxification and is difficult to absorb through the gut, its supplementation is often required to prevent anemia.
- **Lithium** is important for brain function and brain protection, including the potential for promoting the growth of nerve tissue.
- **Magnesium** is one of the most important nutrients in the body. Among its many functions are energy production, activation of vitamins, synthesis of essential molecules (e.g., DNA, RNA, enzymes, and antioxidants), bone and cell membrane structure, and cellular communication.
- **Manganese** is a trace mineral involved in maintaining the health of skin, bone, and cartilage. Additionally, manganese is used by mitochondrial superoxide dismutase to scavenge free radicals, which are abundant in this oxygen-rich organelle. But we don't need a lot of it, whereas the Lyme bacteria is 100 percent dependent on it (see chapter 1).
- **Molybdenum** is a trace mineral that functions as a cofactor for a number of enzymes, including xanthine oxidase, aldehyde oxidase, and sulfite oxidase. Sulfite oxidase is important in the sulfation of various compounds, especially in the brain. This is particularly important, as the brain is often dramatically affected during bouts of toxic exposure.
- **Selenium** is a trace mineral involved in protecting the cell from oxidative damage, particularly in the mitochondria, where it is the cofactor for glutathione peroxidase. Along with other minerals, selenium can help build up white blood cells, enhancing the body's ability to fight illness and infection. High levels of selenium can be toxic; therefore, selenium therapy should be closely monitored. Even when encountering Ebola, one should not exceed 400 µg twice a day.
- **Vanadium** is a trace mineral that is reported[316] to improve blood sugar control and increase muscular strength, as well as improve bone strength.
- **Zinc** is a trace mineral that is vital to many biological functions such as immune resistance, wound healing, digestion, reproduction, physical growth, diabetes control, taste, and smell. More than 300 enzymes in the human body require zinc for proper functioning, including growth and development, the immune response, neurological function, and reproduction.

## GASTROINTESTINAL

Supporting digestion, absorption, and immune function of the GI tract may be just a probiotic away.

- **Beneficial bacteria** (or probiotics) are critical for normal function of the large intestine. Lactobacillus and bifidobacteria, arguably the most important of these bacteria, are used to produce many vitamins and short-chain fatty acids for intestinal health. They also competitively inhibit opportunistic organisms from becoming infectious. It should be noted that some beneficial flora supplements include fructooligosaccharides (FOS). FOS promotes the growth of beneficial flora; however, it may be contraindicated in cases of intestinal yeast overgrowth, as FOS also promotes yeast growth. Beneficial bacterial are commonly deficient in children and adults, especially in those who had limited or no breastfeeding and individuals who have a history of antibiotic treatment.
- **Betaine hydrochloride (HCL)** is commonly referred to as "stomach acid" and is produced and secreted into the stomach in response to the ingestion of protein. HCL is necessary to break down the large structure of proteins, which are further broken down by enzymes in the intestines. Among many possible manifestations, low stomach acid is associated with maldigestion, malabsorption, nutrient deficiencies, reflux disease, and food allergies/sensitivities.
- **Digestive enzymes** are required for normal breakdown of macronutrients (fat, carbohydrates, and protein). Digestive enzyme deficiency results in maldigestion, which manifests similar to HCL deficiency (see above). It is important to differentiate between these two causes of maldigestion and to supplement appropriately.

## ANTIOXIDANTS

These supplements are powerful antioxidants that best fit under this category. Many other supplements listed also have antioxidant activity.

- **Alpha-lipoic acid (ALA)** is a powerful detoxifier and antioxidant. It is used to support detoxification, reduce free-radical load, improve insulin sensitivity, and recycle oxidized glutathione into its reduced (therapeutic) form.
- **Coenzyme Q10 (CoQ10)** is used in every cell of the body for the production of energy and as a powerful antioxidant. It really doesn't matter whether you use the ubiquinone form or ubiquinol.
- **Resveratrol** is a polyphenol compound found in grapes, red wine, purple grape juice, peanuts, and some berries. Resveratrol is a potent

antioxidant: it supports phase 1 and phase 2 detoxification and increases circulation and oxygenation of tissues.

Life Extension Foundation (http://www.lef.org) has high-quality supplements, although they don't carry everything I recommend.

## IMMUNE SUPPORT

Immune support is delivered by providing direct antimicrobial agents, as well as providing immune-stimulating agents.

- **Artemisia** is a natural herbal treatment for infections in the gastrointestinal system, including parasites, bacteria, and yeast. It has anticancer properties, especially when used with HBOT.
- **Candida (yeast) treatments.** Many are afflicted by yeast overgrowth in their intestines, but caprylic acid, oregano oil, garlic, berberine, and artemisia, to name a few, can help. Occasionally, pharmaceutical treatments are needed in the most resistant cases. At the same time, supplements are used that bind up the many toxins that are secreted by yeast during the "die-off" phase, such as bentonite clay.
- **Monolaurin** is a natural monoglyceride found in mother's milk and several medicinal herbs (saw palmetto, bitter melon, etc.). It is known to stimulate immune function, and it possesses antiviral, antifungal, and antibacterial activity while sparing beneficial bacteria found in the gut. It works well with olive leaf extract, which is also antiviral.

## DETOXIFICATION SUPPORT

Detoxification is supported by using supplements that directly detoxify, and by supporting natural detoxification pathways.

- **Alpha-ketoglutarate** is an organic acid involved in the metabolism of amino acids. It is helpful in the elimination of their by-product, ammonia, which is a known neurotoxin.
- **Chlorella** is an alga known to provide naturally occurring nutrition while supporting the removal of toxins such as heavy metals.
- **Epsom salt bath** is magnesium sulfate dissolved into bath water. Magnesium sulfate is absorbed into the circulation and supports normal circulation and detoxification.
- **Indole-3-carbinol (I3C)** is a constituent of cruciferous vegetables and is shown to promote healthy methylation, especially of potentially

harmful hormones. It also helps clean up "bad" estrogens, also known as xenoestrogens. Other names for xenoestrogens are "estrogen mimickers," "hormone imitators," and "endocrine disruptors," such as DDT and glyphosate.

- **Licorice** is an adaptogen, which increases the body's resistance to stress. Two primary physiologic functions of licorice include conserving cortisol, an important adrenal hormone, and healing the mucosal lining of the digestive tract. Licorice also supports liver function and detoxification and supports the synergy of other herbal medications.

## VITAMINS

Vitamins may be required at higher levels because of genetic predispositions and because of increased burden on the body:

- **Folinic acid,** also known as L-5-methyl tetrahydrofolate, is an active form of folic acid. It is used in folate deficiency and impaired methylation, and especially in individuals with the MTHFR genetic predisposition.
- **Methylcobalamine (methyl-B$_{12}$)** is the active form of vitamin B$_{12}$, which plays an important role in the health of red blood cells. It is used as a treatment for megaloblastic anemia. It is also important for methylation reactions and immune system regulation. Methylcobalamine acts as a methyl donor and participates in the synthesis of SAM-e (S-adenosylmethionine), a nutrient that has powerful mood-stabilizing properties. Those with a double COMT mutation should strive to use hydroxy-cobalamine.
- **Pyridoxal-5-phosphate (P5P)** is the activated form of pyridoxine (vitamin B$_6$). P5P is the cofactor for many enzymatic reactions within the body, the most important being in amino acid metabolism. In particular, methylation reactions are dependent on P5P, which play a central role in detoxification and brain chemistry. Also, the activation of B$_6$ requires adequate availability of magnesium, which is found to be insufficient in many individuals. Supplementing P5P provides activated B$_6$ directly. Vitamin B$_6$ (and P5P) may be contraindicated in cases of intestinal yeast overgrowth, as it can promote yeast growth.
- **Vitamin A** is a fat-soluble vitamin that is a potent immune stimulator, which is helpful at higher doses for fighting infections (especially measles). Since vitamin A is a fat-soluble vitamin, eliminating excessive amounts of it is much more difficult than with water-soluble vitamins (e.g., vitamins B and C). As a result, excessive ingestion or supplementation

of vitamin A can be toxic—just an FYI. Don't take large doses for long periods like you can with vitamin $D_3$.

- **Vitamin C** is one of the most potent water-soluble antioxidants. In addition to its antioxidant benefit, vitamin C is involved in many biologic functions, including antihistaminic activity, immune function support, and the production of carnitine and brain chemicals.
- **Vitamin D** is a fat-soluble vitamin most notably involved in the healthy metabolism of calcium for normal bone development. It is also associated with many physiologic functions, including enhancing innate immunity and inhibiting the development of autoimmunity.
- **Vitamin E** is a fat-soluble vitamin predominately used as an antioxidant. Vitamin E is also capable of thinning the blood and supporting immune function.
- **Vitamin K** is most commonly associated with facilitating the clotting cascade; however, vitamin K is also a potent antioxidant and anti-inflammatory (IL-6) inhibitor and is involved in the development of the nervous system. Vitamin K deficiency may also be associated with uncontrolled neuronal firing that presents as neurological symptoms.

## MISCELLANEOUS

- **Essential fatty acids (EFAs)** are primarily omega-3 and DHA. These well-studied fats are shown to be anti-inflammatory, immune-stimulating, and hypoallergenic. They also help thin the blood to increase circulation and are used for the healthy development of brain tissue.
- **Inositol hexaphosphate (IP6)** supports normal cell growth and development through its role in cellular signaling and support of natural cell defense.
- **Melatonin**, a hormone secreted by the pineal gland, is most popularly associated with promoting restful sleep. Additionally, melatonin has antioxidant activity and may prevent damage to the brain, as well as promoting learning and memory in individuals with neurode generation.
- **Ribose** is a necessary substrate for synthesis of nucleotides, and it is a part of the building blocks that form DNA and RNA molecules. Among many benefits, ribose has been shown[317] to improve quality of sleep, energy, and cognitive function.
- **Oxytocin** is a hormone that blocks inappropriate panic and fear from entering the limbic system or emotional centers of the brain. It stimulates brain growth in the social centers in the brain.
- **A-10/ phenyl butyrate** is an orphan drug. Its metabolites demethylate DNA and turn back on genes that have inappropriately been turned

off (such as cancer suppressor genes).[318] We know there are genes in the brains of children on the spectrum that have been inappropriately turned off. Cancer patients often have their cancer suppressor genes turned off. A-10 is not a prescription and can be taken orally, but PB can be given only as in IV. Anyone who has suffered through a chronic illness could benefit from having his or her DNA demethyalted.

## TREATMENT RATIONALE

The term "toxin" refers to a host of agents, from heavy metals and organic pollutants to infectious agents, electrical pollutants, and ionizing radiation. We know what they are: glyphosate, HH-DNA (homologus human DNA) found in vaccines, viral contaminants in vaccines, and mid-weight metals, such as aluminum.

The term "detoxification" refers to the direct removal of toxins, or inactivation of a toxin's detrimental effect.

Worldwide, we are inundated with an incredible number of toxic substances. In the United States there are over 80,000 recorded chemicals in use, with 4 billion pounds of chemicals released into the environment, including 72 million pounds of known carcinogens. Sadly, we know very little about the effects of these substances on a developing brain. Only a dozen or so chemicals have been tested for neurotoxicity, including mercury, lead, PCBs, Roundup, alcohol, nicotine, and a few pesticides, especially DDT/DDE and dicofol.

The trend is clear: a host of diseases and symptoms are now commonplace, but the underlying cause is largely going unnoticed. With greater amounts of toxins in our environment, we will continue to accumulate more of these toxins in our bodies.

When we start off with toxins from before birth, and begin to accumulate toxins immediately after birth, we can expect disease to manifest if protective and detoxification mechanisms are impaired.

Children on the autism spectrum who are exposed to mercury in utero are commonly unable to excrete mercury—even when intravenous glutathione is administered—until nutritional deficiencies are corrected.

Although many toxins may be incorporated into an individual, these toxins may not become manifest in symptoms or disease until a critical threshold is exceeded. An individual's threshold or "tipping point" is determined by several factors, including genetic predispositions and nutritional sufficiency, which are identified as biomarkers of susceptibility.

Our bodies handle all toxins through a two-step process, called phase I and phase II detoxification (also described in chapter 2). Phase I involves the biotransformation of toxic agents using the cytochrome P-450 system in the liver. This is a mixed-function enzyme system that converts toxins via oxidation/reduction and hydrolysis. The objectives of phase I are to make toxins more water-soluble for elimination and to prepare them for further processing in phase II.

Phase II involves peptide conjugation, which is heavily dependent upon amino acids derived from dietary proteins. Genetic defects in the production or utilization of these peptides, such as impaired sulfation or glutathione conjugation, can impair phase II detoxification. Digestive enzyme deficiencies and/or low stomach acid can impair protein digestion and contribute to amino acid deficiency. Any stress, including toxic and emotional stressors, can result in impaired enzyme production, leading to amino acid deficiency and impaired phase II; this results in the individual having a blocked phase II and impaired elimination of toxins.

Also, undigested proteins can induce growth of abnormal intestinal bacteria and yeast, resulting in an increased production of microbial-derived toxins. These toxins can irritate or paralyze the gut and produce a host of foul aromatic compounds that are frequently described by parents of autistic children. These toxins also may induce inflammation and swelling of the intestinal wall, leading to an impaired gut barrier and subsequent absorption of undigested proteins that commonly provoke food allergies and other various allergic reactions.

Immune cells in the intestinal tract are designed to protect against any invading organism. However, the presence of foreign proteins and other toxins can overwhelm the immune system's ability to respond effectively, increasing susceptibility to infection and autoimmunity.

Effective phase I and II (detoxification) processing is needed for adequate removal of the many toxins we are exposed to in our environment. Adequate oxygen, exercise, and dietary nutrition generally results in normal functioning of phase I and II. Moderate exercise can be used to enhance insufficient phase I and II detoxification pathways.

Problems arise when an individual has blocked detoxification pathways, but the toxins themselves can block these pathways. This interference also occurs frequently during normal physiologic processes, such as the stress response, which can impair digestive function. Treatments to enhance phase I include therapies such as hyperbaric oxygen therapy (HBOT) and hot or infrared saunas. These modalities particularly mobilize organic pollutants, which increases the requirement for nutrient cofactors and phase II activity.

Impaired phase II can result in the accumulation of oxidative intermediates that may be more damaging than the original toxin. This type of response can result from pushing phase I modalities when phase II is blocked. As stated previously, phase II is heavily dependent on having good bowel and digestive function to support elimination. Without good bowel and digestive function, pushing phase II, as with any type of detoxification therapy, can result in adverse reactions. Therapies for improving bile flow and bowel function should be used prior to pushing phase II modalities. Supporting regular bowel movements and using non-absorbable agents that bind toxins in the gastrointestinal track prior to phase II treatments can help prevent toxic reactions.

Few of us realize our bodies are electrical, but the heart and brain and even lungs are electrical. Exposure to electric fields and ionizing radiation magnifies the effect of other toxins in the body, and vice versa. This magnifying effect is particularly true when toxins contain an electric charge, like heavy metals.

Electrostatic charges in the atmosphere can increase toxic exposure, as these attract charged particles, in particular heavy metals, into the area. Acidifying pollutants, such as aluminum, sulfur dioxide ($SO_2$), nitrogen oxides (NO), and ammonia ($NH_3$), which are especially high in industrialized areas, also attract and increase the atmospheric deposition of heavy metals such as mercury.

The arrival of mercury-free/trace mercury vaccines in the United States was obscured by the fact that other exposures to mercury have increased. Atmospheric and dietary mercury, to name a few, have increased, and mothers during pregnancy contain higher levels of mercury as well.

The goals are reducing toxic burden, improving detoxification capabilities, restoring gut function, addressing low-grade infections and immune dysfunction, and providing nutritional supplementation.

## A SPECIAL WORD ON HEAVY METALS

There is politics in every human endeavor, and no less so in medicine. Louis Pasteur couldn't publish his work on pasteurization in the beer- and wine-making processes because everyone "knew" that yeast was an inert ingredient in brewing. Thus he published on spoiled milk instead and became famous for pasteurizing milk. Ignaz Semmelweiss, a Hungarian OB-GYN, was discredited, imprisoned, and died for having the audacity to insist that physicians wash their hands before delivering babies. The same level of politics and blindness exists today.

When it comes to heavy metals, some might say, "If removing heavy metals worked as a treatment for children and adults susceptible to heavy-metal poisoning, everyone would be doing it." But if one thing should be clear from reading this book, environmental issues are rarely explored as a treatment for anything. Environmental medicine is not taught in medical school, probably by design.

Mercury is the second deadliest neurotoxin known to man, and the CDC's own Agency for Toxic Substances and Disease Registry (ATSDR) has thousands of references in the scientific literature showing it causes neurological disorders, heart attacks, stroke, and even cancer. The CDC took mercury out of indoor paint two decades ago when two children in a single family died, but it seems to turn a blind eye (greased-palm eye) when it comes to mercury in vaccines, and yes . . . there is still mercury in certain vaccines given in the United States.

## MERCURY AMALGAM REMOVAL INSTRUCTIONS FOR ADULTS

Many children and adults still have and receive mercury laden dental fillings called silver or mercury amalgam fillings. It is best not to get one but if you have them it is best to remove them.

1. For two weeks prior to having dental amalgams, eat a diet high in proteins and vegetables.
2. Ensure that you have one to two bowel movements per day. Magnesium citrate suspension can be added to water, tea, or juice, one or two tablespoons per day to induce the two bowel movements. Be sure to drink lots of water, about half of your weight in ounces per day, divided over your waking hours on a daily basis, such as four ounces or a cup of drinking water each hour that you are awake. You can also add ground or powdered flaxseed to your drinks or foods like sauces or cereals or salads (one or two heaping tablespoons per day) to induce two bowel movements per day.

3. For three days prior to the amalgams being removed, take
   * Chlorella, 1 gram three times a day
   * Vitamin C, 1 gram three times a day
   * Cilantro, 1 gram three times a day
   * Glutathione 3,000 mg (bonus to take garlic with this as well)
4. Right before going to the dentist, take 3,000 mg (3 g) of chlorella and 3,000 mg (3 g) of vitamin C.
5. The dentist should provide you with a source of oxygen by mask or nasal cannula so that you do not breathe in the toxic gas that comes out of your mouth as he or she drills out the amalgam filling. The dentist should also use a coarse bit that breaks up the amalgam into chunks, rather than a fine bit that pulverizes the amalgam, which can spread and penetrate more easily. She should use a high-volume suction apparatus and a rubber dam to reduce your exposure to the toxic particulates.
6. Chlorella dissolved in the rinse water and sprayed in the mouth helps further reduce exposure during the procedure. Eye protection is also provided to the patient to avoid exposure through the conjunctiva. The dentist and her assistant should use a gas mask and eye protection to protect themselves from the toxic fumes, and the procedure should be performed in a room that does not have air circulated

around in the office. The air in the room should be vented separately, with appropriate filtration to trap the mercury released from the drilling. An anionic air-purifying device in the room may also be helpful. The dentist should use a lot of water and chlorella rinse and spray to bind the mercury to reduce exposure.

7. Only one quadrant or less should be removed at a time unless the fillings are small, based on the dentist's preference and experience. After the procedure, do the procedures listed in number 4 for an additional three days. Reduce doses prescribed by one-half for child less than 100 pounds.

## FREQUENT, LOW-DOSE ORAL CHELATION

Getting rid of heavy metals has implication for patients who have diabetes and are at risk for cardiovascular disease. It is not just for people who eat a lot of fish or have had amalgams in their mouths. The next step up from chlorella and cilantro is a program first developed by Andrew Hall Cutler, PhD, and a chemist who found himself poisoned by his mercury amalgams.

Children have been safely treated with his protocol for many years. Of course, chelation can be a dangerous act if done improperly. "Improperly" would be dosing a chelator higher than one's body can eliminate, or dosing for only a short period of time, which raises the risk of redistribution.

Andy Cutler used the half-lives of the chelating agent to devise his protocol. So, his method uses low, frequent doses given continuously, so as to not risk redistribution after every dose.

The chelators selected by Dr. Cutler for chelation are DMSA and ALA (alpha-lipoic acid). ALA is taken every three hours around the clock, DMSA every four hours.

The chelators are taken for seventy-two hours. Every period of three days is called a "round," and every round is followed by a break of at least equal time (3+ days).

DMSA, or dimercaptosuccinic acid, is an organic compound that contains sulfur. DMSA can also cause deficiencies of several minerals, such as molybdenum and zinc. So you have to supplement these minerals even if they are in your multivitamin.

Adrenal fatigue is another common issue in detoxification. If you notice labile emotions for no apparent reason (yeast), think adrenals (licorice, P5P, pantothenic acid, lavender, skullcap, and ginseng).

## HELPFUL SUPPLEMENTS FOR CHELATION

The following should be given three to four times per day:

- Vitamin C: 500 to 1,000 mg/day divided into four doses
- Magnesium: 400 mg/day per day divided into four doses
- Zinc: 30 to 50 mg/day divided into four doses
- Fat-soluble supplements given once per day
- Vitamin E: 400 IU/day (d-alpha tocopherol, not dl-alpha tocopherol)
- Molybdenum: Sulphites are also found in many foods and must be converted to nontoxic sulphates by the liver, which requires an enzyme called sulphite oxidase (SO) which requires molybdenum. Mercury can substitute itself for molybdenum, rendering the enzyme useless, making molybdenum an important mineral to take while chelating, especially those with high copper as molybdenum reduces copper absorption. ALA tends to increase copper retention and molybdenum will help a lot when ALA is being used.

## DOSING THE CHELATORS: SLOW AND STEADY WINS THE RACE

If there has been no exposure to mercury within the past three months (vaccines, a broken CFL bulb, amalgams), you can start with DMSA or ALA.

If there has been a recent exposure:
- Use DMSA first and for a couple of months before you introduce ALA.
- Begin dosing with either 1/8th mg per pound or even lower 1/10th to 1/16th of both the DMSA and ALA (don't add in the ALA initially). You can work up to 1/2 mg per pound slowly over time, but in no case should an increase be greater than 50 percent, and at least five rounds at each dose should be completed.

The chelators are given around the clock:
- DMSA every three to four hours
- ALA every three hours
- For three days. Optional: ALA can be given every four hours for two stretches during the night to accommodate the sleep schedule only. The body metabolizes more slowly at night. Please don't wake up yourself or anyone else more than once per night.

### Missed Doses

I know Cutler would have people stop a round if a dose is skipped or late, but I don't think that should be necessary. Stay on track but don't get bent out of shape because you can't exactly follow a tight schedule.

Chelators can be given at closer intervals (two hours; forty-five minutes; etc.) but stay on track if possible.

## HOW LONG DOES CHELATION TAKE?

Chelation often takes between 100 to 300 rounds. Slow and steady wins the race! If you have been having symptoms of mercury toxicity, the improvements you will experience should be enough to keep you on track.

# 9

# The End of Addiction? (New for Revised Edition)

*As you read in the original introduction, I briefly eluded to a protocol I have been using to treat addictions and specifically alcoholism. But in the first edition I did not elaborate, which I regretted, but herewith make up for what should have been in the first edition.*

Alcoholism affects more than 27 million Americans. In a world where less than 10 percent of those with alcohol addiction are getting treatment, note that most know how to treat Alcohol Use Disorder (AUD). First and foremost, should anyone discover an efficient way to treat alcoholism that doesn't make Big Pharma money, you won't hear about it (PERIOD).

One of my interests in the chemistry of alcohol addiction stems from my own personal inability to get an endorphin release from drinking alcohol. It will make me sleepy, but there is no other secondary gain for me. I obviously was not experiencing what others were experiencing, and I attempted to figure it all out.

## SUBOXONE

Addiction medicine hasn't changed for a long time with the exception of the introduction of Suboxone—an opioid buprenorphine in combination with naloxone. Naloxone, frequently referred to as Narcan, is an opioid receptor antagonist that effectively occupies the human opioid receptors, but blocks any action. Suboxone is one of the primary pharmaceuticals used today in medication-assisted therapy (MAT) for opiate addiction.

Suboxone obviously helps with the neurotransmitter aspects of an opioid addiction, because it is an opioid that provides a short-term fix that makes it easier to adapt to long-term treatment. If one is choosing between Suboxone and doing nothing, then Suboxone is a better choice. But it is not real addiction treatment for opioid addiction, let alone any other kind of addiction.

The process of addiction—and the underlying disorder addiction mitigates—is the actual problem. Opioids, nicotine, cocaine, or alcohol are ultimately a form of self-medication—just the means to an end.

## NALTREXONE AND THE SINCLAIR METHOD

Naltrexone is a treatment option that was introduced in the 1960s and is used in the Sinclair method as a stand-alone drug for alcohol addiction treatment. The medication reduces opioid effects by competing for opiate receptors and displacing opioid drugs from these receptors, reversing their effects. The metabolite of naltrexone, 6β-naltrexol, is also an active agonist. Consequently, the effects of naltrexone arise from both the parent drug and its major metabolite and last about a day. It is capable of antagonizing all four types of opiate receptors.

AUD patients prescribed naltrexone take the medication orally about an hour (and only then) before drinking, blocking the positive-reinforcement effects of alcohol, which allows the person to stop or reduce drinking (the Sinclair method). This occurs because for an alcohol addict, drinking causes a massive release of dopamine and endorphins, the source of intense craving for alcohol, even years after being sober. Alcohol also increases the activity of GABA (γ-aminobutyric acid), a major inhibitory neurotransmitter in the brain that suppresses activity of the central nervous system with accompanying calmative effects.

This opioid blocker is intended to reduce and eventually erase habit-forming behaviors, diminishing a person's craving for alcohol to its pre-addiction state. This assumes that the primary underlying dynamics in alcohol addiction are habit and conditioned response. However, the limited success of naltrexone alone makes it clear that more complex neurochemical and genetic factors are involved.

Naltrexone and naloxone differ in their utility in addiction treatment. Naloxone is effective in opioid overdose rescues, acting within minutes to reduce opioid levels, which lasts for about an hour because of rapid metabolism. The different half-lives of naltrexone and naloxone explain why the two drugs have different purposes. Naltrexone is used to block cravings for both opioids and alcohol but naloxone is not, while naloxone can treat overdoses but naltrexone cannot. Both drugs block the analgesic action of both exogenous opioids and the pleasure response of endogenous endorphins, but naloxone acts quickly enough to treat an overdose, while naltrexone does not. For these same reasons, naltrexone cannot be used to rescue someone from an overdose, but can be used to help people who are addicted to opioids have less craving for them.

However, I have never used naltrexone to treat addictions. Rather, I use the bio-identical hormone oxytocin to achieve the same effect, because it also sits on the body's opioid receptors, is capable of putting opioid addicts into withdrawal, and has agonist action comparable to naltrexone.

## OXYTOCIN

No one, as far as I know, has compared oxytocin to naltrexone, but naltrexone is considered only modestly successful at treating AUD, and oxytocin by itself has had only modest success in my clinical experience. Consequently, I do not use oxytocin alone for AUD, because it does not get the job done. Modest success is not satisfactory.

Initially, I started using oxytocin because it helped my brain-injured patients deal with the Post-Traumatic Stress Disorder (PTSD) that comes along for free when one has a stroke, TBI, or some other form of brain injury. As the brain heals and one becomes more aware of how messed up life is, that can cause a great of anger and anxiety ... the oxytocin blocks inappropriate fear and panic from engaging the limbic area of the brain. It even seems to help the brain process more effectively. When I learned that one of the effects of drinking alcohol is to increase oxytocin levels, I thought it was worth a trial to use it in alcohol cessation. However, while oxytocin may be a secondary gain from drinking alcohol, oxytocin-seeking is not the driving mechanism of the addiction.

Rather, I believe that the ultimate hook in alcoholism is the endorphin explosion that those prone to addiction experience. Without this endorphin explosion in individuals with the wrong constitution or genetics, there would be no craving and no addiction.

## BACLOFEN

This brings us to the classic drug baclofen. Without getting too technical, the meso-corticolimbic (MCL) dopamine (DA) system plays a critical role in mediating the positive reinforcing effects of a variety of abused drugs, including cocaine, amphetamine, nicotine, and opiates.[319, 320, 321] This anatomical pathway originates from the ventral tegmental area (VTA) in the midbrain and projects to several forebrain regions, including the nucleus accumbens (NAcc) and medial prefrontal cortex (mPFC).[322]

Since opiate receptor activation generally inhibits individual neurons, opiate-induced DA release was initially hypothesized to be mediated by a disinhibitory mechanism, i.e. opiates inhibit VTA GABAergic interneurons to decrease GABA release, which subsequently disinhibits VTA DA neurons, leading to an increase in NAcc DA release.[323] The mesolimbic DA system may be the substrate upon which opiates act to produce their reinforcing effects.[324] One could then postulate that if GABA is provided in therapeutic amounts, the VTA DA neurons will not become disinhibited.

Baclofen has already distinguished itself in the medical literature for utility in treating AUD (when the dose is allowed to be titrated up to whatever level a patient needs to obtain control). This point bears repeating because the medical literature is replete with randomized trials showing that baclofen does not work, but when you consider the dose used in the trials, it was inadequate. It is only when the patient is allowed to slowly titrate the dose up without limit that one sees the desired effect.[325] Be that as it may, the mixed results from studies with suboptimal doses have stifled baclofen's utilization for treating addictions, specifically in AUD. A double-blind RCT using baclofen for cigarette cessation published in 2015 was successful at 20 mg four times a day.[326] Still, that dose is usually far too low for AUD. The logistical issue is that there are very few physicians who will give an AUD patient the opportunity to try baclofen, because they have no training in using it for AUD, let alone using it with potentially high-dose titration. It is noteworthy that not all AUD patients need high dose levels, but many do. This all makes sense if you understand that as a GABA agonist, baclofen seems to prevent the disinhibition of the VTA DA neurons (i.e. inhibiting dopamine production), so there is no reinforcement for the addictive behavior.

## CBD

This brings us to CBD. Discrete disturbances of AMPA GluR1 and cannabinoid type-1 receptor expression, observed in the NAcc, associated with stimulus cue-induced heroin-seeking, were normalized by CBD treatment.[327] CBDs can be initiated at full dose out of the starting gate—there is no need to wait to bring up the baclofen dose to therapeutic levels (however long that takes). Between baclofen and CBD, the VTA DA neurons remain inhibited and oxytocin is just icing on the cake—the endorphin cake—by inhibiting a release that would only serve to reinforce the addictive behavior and by supporting a sense of wellbeing.

## PROTOCOL

These three relatively benign medications in tandem support an affordable, effective intervention in which the mechanisms for eliminating addiction reinforcement are relatively well-understood and well-documented.

- Baclofen
  *Initial titration*. I start patients off at a very low dosage of baclofen, because some people are very sensitive, so we begin at 5 mg twice a day. I have them slowly increase their dose to 20 mg QID (four times a day). This is the dosage that was used in the cigarette trial. One has to increase

the dose slowly while the patient acclimates to the somnambulistic quality of baclofen. However, as pointed out, that dose is usually inadequate for AUD.

*Caution in weaning.* It is also important to wean off the baclofen slowly. This is absolutely not a drug that can be quit cold turkey. Reported potential side effects of abrupt weaning include hallucinations and seizures.[328]

- **CBD.** The required dose of CBD is 40 mg QID (four times a day).
- **Oxytocin.** The oxytocin cannot be used until the patient is sober, because that will put people with opioid addiction into withdrawal. Once they are sober, sublingual troches of 25 mg of oxytocin, used up to four times a day, complete the protocol.
- **Contraindications.** Note that oxytocin cannot be given to pregnant women. Patients with brain injuries, stealth brain infections such as Lyme or cytomegalovirus, or severe dementia may not be good candidates for this protocol.

Nothing works 100 percent of the time on 100 percent of people. For the majority of patients, this protocol has great potential and is relatively inexpensive. Oxytocin 25 mg troches can be purchased (via compounding pharmacies) for less than a dollar/day in most cases, so perhaps $3/day at maximum dosage. CBD can vary widely in price, but a fair price is $60 for an ounce tincture in which one drop is 1 mg, so at maximum dose, the cost is $120 per week. Baclofen is sold for pennies a tablet. The cost is about $500 per month for this protocol. How long anyone stays on the protocol is between him or her and their physician.

Addiction management is ultimately very individualized. If the patient needs a high dose of baclofen, it can take a couple of months to ramp up the dose to a helpful level. While I let folks wean themselves off baclofen when they no longer need it, I encourage them to take the CBD and oxytocin ongoing. These are benign calmatives. Additionally, the patient can always reintroduce the baclofen if they need it.

While naltrexone, used in the Sinclair Method, is only $50 a month if insurance is covering the medication, in my experience it does not work for everyone. While the naltrexone prevents the endorphin explosion after drinking, it does not help brain processes that are mitigated by oxytocin.

Naltrexone also does not deal with the ongoing cravings (psychological) that many experience for a lifetime afterward, even after years of sobriety. The naltrexone only blocks secondary gain (dopamine and endorphin release) at the moment of imbibing. Additionally, naltrexone is not effective for addiction to cigarettes, cocaine, or other substances. Those prone to addiction get addicted to all sorts of things. Ultimately it is the underlying addiction chemistry itself that we need to address.

Addiction treatment using Suboxone can take two years, serving as a bridge while one is doing other things in their life to cope with the addiction. The medication often only works when it is taken consistently. It doesn't really move the gauge, just keeps the gauge from going into the red zone.

To date, no one has published on the clinical use of baclofen and CBD in combination with oxytocin for addiction mitigation. Nevertheless, I do not expect that what I just revealed will change the face of addiction medicine. In fact, it is not a problem limited to addiction medicine; it is ubiquitous through the entire medical paradigm. If a medication or an intervention is not going to make a profit for a corporation that can adequately promote, market, and educate the medical community, no one is going to hear about it, let alone use it.

Pharma companies will sit on useful medical knowledge they could share, but do not share, because they either will not profit from it or because that knowledge will interfere with the marketing of something they want sold. The corporate control of medicine is so endemic, most physicians have no idea their clinical choices are controlled and truncated by corporations, not science. Well, maybe they have a better idea now post-COVID. Pharma was not shy about marginalizing, minimizing, and censoring any physician that was objecting to their narratives.

# Conclusion

*"There have been, and will be again, many destructions of mankind arising out of many causes."*

—Plato, *Timaeus/Critias*

Over one-half of US children currently have at least one chronic health condition. It seems to be human nature to let things get so bad that something has to become a dire emergency before corrective action is taken. Yet we are well past dire emergency and nothing is being done because others are running interference. If the current trend is not altered by 2025, one-half of children in the US are projected to have what is called *autism* (an environmentally triggered brain injury). Is this by design? Is this about accelerating the collapse of the experiment called the United States?

It seems so cliché to point out that our government is massively corrupt because of the vast sums of money we allow into politics. This will eventually run its course as it is simply not sustainable, but it seems to be running its course in a very unconscious way, which is never a positive. Unfortunately, many that understand this are not here to help but to profit. It is no secret how to bring down an empire. There are those who are preparing right now to take financial and political advantage of doing just that. By stealth, by deception, by corruption we have let a few control healthcare for their own benefit.

The book you have just read is not the only voice delivering a vital message we all need to get wise to. On the cusp of 2016, an article was published entitled "The Subversion of Medicine and Public Health by International Security Prerogatives."[329]

Medicine and public health are compromised by the highest echelons of science, industry and public administration for the geopolitical objectives of international cohabitation, preservation of resources, environmental conservation and decarbonization, all of which hinge on depopulation. Under the cover of reproductive health involuntary sterilizations are implemented throughout the developing world through adulterated vaccines while in the developed world flu immunization programs weaken the immune systems of the old and civil servants to shorten lifespans and spare governments from meeting insolvent healthcare and pension plan obligations in the last stage of the demographic transition. Endocrine disruptors inserted in the basic elements of life to presumably prevent caries chronically subvert the human reproductive system to lower the total fertility rate of every country to replacement level. In the name of sustainable development, experimental carbon capture and sequestration methods as well as solar radiation management methods double as weapons against longevity by subjecting billions to unnaturally high exposure levels of heavy metals so the world's decarbonization goals are tackled from two directions, by reducing greenhouse gases in the atmosphere and increasing morbidity and mortality among the general population to proactively lower future emissions. Poverty and hunger are used as fronts for the deployment of GMO crops that purportedly increase yields, improve nutrition and require fewer fertilizers and pesticides, but that in fact misuse the latest bioengineering advances to cause subfertility, immune deficiencies and crop failures and thus lower the population by limiting births and increasing deaths. Unless stopped, this engineered genocide will damage the genetic and intellectual endowment of humanity and cause population collapse within 20 years, time during which the incidence and severity of NCDs will grow exponentially irrespective of health system investments and medical breakthroughs. Only a political solution can restore our health as individuals and as a civilization.

## THE ROMAN EMPIRE

At its zenith, the Roman Empire stretched from Loch Ness to the pyramids at Giza. Imperial Rome lasted half a millennium until "barbarians" and pirates invaded Italy throughout the fifth century AD. Rome, a city of millions, became a mere town of a few thousand, and the Dark Ages were upon Western civilization. It is never just one thing . . . lead in the water didn't help, food shortages perhaps, but what most likely brought it all down was something very, very small—the mosquitoes that arrived from Africa with malaria at the dawn of the common era. If mosquitoes are being used today for something nefarious, it is being done by those that know their history.

Today we have fluoride in our water, not lead, but fluoride is more toxic than lead. We have pesticides sprayed on our food and other nastiness sprayed from the skies for "geoengineering." We have mandated vaccines containing several heavy metals and contaminated with cancer-causing retroviruses. The American Empire has spread itself around the globe, its resources diverted into the military-industrial complex and a central government under the control of global banks, corporations, and the very few families who control them. This isn't the 1 percent; this is the 0.000066 percent. Whether you call them Spectre, Hydra, the Illuminati, or Brothers of the Shadow, it matters not. What matters is that we have let them get away with this.

Malaria is not the problem in the United States, but the *Borrelia* class of organisms is (coming primarily from tick bites infecting at least 50 million Americans, most of whom will never know what brought them to their knees). Then there is the out-of-control destruction of the future unless we stop the mass poisoning. Collapse of institutions, collapse of the economy, and collapse of society, as we know it, is probably already inevitable because the status quo isn't any more sustainable than what took place with the Roman Empire. Unlike the Roman Empire, today there is this 0.000066 percent who think they will be able to control and profit from the event that they are maneuvering into place.

Plato would have us believe that there was once an advanced civilization in the Atlantic beyond the Pillars of Hercules. There is no official confirmation of his story, but then official reports are often less than truthful. The issue is not whether the story is credible or not; the issue is the archetype in the story Plato told.

## FROM ATLANTIS TO UTERUS

The archetype is that of having everything and then losing everything, and that archetype is being played out today in so many ways. If there was an Atlantis, its destruction may have taken place well over 12,000 years ago, but to bring this back to the modern era and return to medicine, I will take you back only forty-some years when I remember reading a full-page ad in a medical throwaway newspaper in which some pharmaceutical corporate entity said they were reserving the Nobel Prize (not something in their power) for the person who came up with the cure for preeclampsia/eclampsia.

Preeclampsia (PE) is a disorder characterized by high blood pressure and a large amount of protein in the urine, which most often occurs in the third trimester of pregnancy and can evolve into the life-threatening form called eclampsia.

The official medical cause of PE and E is that it is a mystery (of course), but it has been known for years that this is a nutritional issue (malnutrition).[330] Without getting into too much detail, it seems that if women have mutations in the genes that service the methylation cycle in their bodies, such as the methylenetetrahydrofolate reductase (MTHFR)[331] gene, then they are definitely more prone to get this disorder. The preventive treatment would not only include magnesium, which has been found to be so useful in the treatment of severe PE and E, but also an assortment of vitamins and minerals that would support women who have metabolic issues and malnutrition either because of these polymorphisms or because their diets are inadequate. That means magnesium, zinc, vitamin B$_6$, biologically active B$_9$—such as folinic acid—and several antioxidants, along with a good foundation of other B vitamins.

Just giving oral magnesium alone would be an easy and simple fix, but it won't do the job. Remember: we are talking about women who are malnourished, so you don't just supplement with one thing and expect it to do the job, even though giving it intravenously has been found to be so helpful. They are malnourished because they are most likely eating standard American diet.

The take-home message here is twofold: first, MDs (conventionally trained physicians) know almost nothing about nutrition. When I went to medical school, only 20 percent of schools had a course in nutrition, and the average length of that course was two hours. This lack of knowledge about the importance of nutrition and the nutritional knowledge that a physician should have is missing by design.

In fact, many physicians (MDs/DOs) reading the above two paragraphs will find a discussion about MTFHR and the methylation cycle difficult to understand—this is simply not the language they speak. They will say their patients aren't malnourished when they haven't the foggiest idea what being nourished means. Being malnourished doesn't mean you look like a concentration camp survivor (that is being starved and malnourished).

The second message is about understanding how we got in this mess. One hundred years ago, the Rockefeller Foundation propaganda Flexner Report made it impossible for medical schools to exist that were competing with pharmaceutical-oriented schools (allopathic medicine) supported by the Rockefeller Foundation. They also wanted to control what physicians were taught. It was important for physicians not to have any knowledge that might either interfere with the sale of patentable medicines or a better way to treat without patentable drugs.

## THE BIRTH OF BIG PHARMA

Rockefeller wanted to control the market for his drug and pharmaceutical industries. However, first he had to get rid of the competition, and so all schools teaching naturopathy, homeopathy, and eclectic medicine were destroyed. It also meant getting rid of anything natural that might be better than the drugs they wanted to push, so cannabis/hemp, for example, had to become illegal. Thus Big Pharma was born!

This piece of history has to be understood to know why today we have very expensive "bandage" care instead of healthcare. For food, we have poisoned slop from the corporations that have seized food production and drenched it in pesticides. Why are so many of the highly intelligent men and women in conventional medicine so unhappy with their profession even as most are still oblivious to the undue influence they are under?

The controlled media periodically gets interested in contaminated Tylenol but has no concern for the stuff Tylenol is made of—acetaminophen depletes glutathione from the liver, rendering it more vulnerable to toxic damage, and it damages the kidneys, just like thimerosol does. There are about 16,000 deaths each year in the United States from prescription painkillers. What do you want to bet that is from the acetaminophen that gets piggybacked on the narcotic? The media seems to relish in panicking us over a few cases of measles but says nothing about the MMR vaccine itself being a worthless intervention that has serious side effects. It is because they are *bought*.

We have an illegal drug problem in our country because factions of the government wanted there to be a drug problem and were never held accountable—and are not being held accountable. Drug trafficking has always been a sure-thing fund-raiser for the deep government in order to finance black-ops, and if it could target certain undesirable ethnic populations, all the better. This is not ancient history, such as the stories Gary Webb reported on in the summer of 1996 in the *San Jose Mercury News*. In it, he reported that a drug ring that sold millions of dollars worth of cocaine in Los Angeles was funneling its profits to the CIA's army in Nicaragua, known as the Contras.[332] Are we to believe this still isn't going on?

But you don't have to be involved in some clandestine operation to be screwing over people with drugs ("U.S. Maker of OxyContin painkiller to pay $600 million in guilty plea" [2007, *The New York Times*, Barry Meier]). Nice: Purdue Pharma trained its sales representatives to make deceptive statements by telling doctors that the drug was less likely to be abused, but the sales representatives also gave false information about the risks of opioid withdrawal after stopping the pill. Between 1996 and 2001 alone, Purdue made almost $3 billion on this drug. The fine of $600 million is 0.3 percent of what they made selling the drug in just that five-year period. Sounds like the cost of doing business to me, and a fairly minor cost.

I have come down hard on my colleagues. You don't read the medical literature, but maybe one of the reasons they don't is that a lot of research is fabricated. And if you don't know what to believe, you may read nothing.

Three billion dollars a year are spent on direct-to-consumer ads, but that doesn't include the money pharmaceutical companies will spend influencing prescription practices, be they in academic or in clinical medicine; and they know which physicians to target and who sets the trends. They know which politicians to target as well.

Did you know that a decade ago, when statin drugs came on the scene, like lard in a pigpen, it was in part due to the fact that over 90 percent of the physicians[333] who wrote those guidelines were on the "take" (baksheesh)?

So, although practicing physicians don't read the medical literature, I can tell you they do read the guidelines written by venerated academic physicians, and opinion pieces in major medical journals. Have these people all been bought off?

That is how we end up with medicines that kill instead of heal. First the academicians are bought, such as department chairmen. Then pharmaceutical companies or front groups for the CDC will endow special academic chairs (faculty positions) for their moles (penetration agents) and mouthpieces (Paul Offit probably being the most recognized of those who would fall in this category). Then they bleed out the federal agencies themselves like the CDC, the FDA, the EPA, and the USDA, and then the courts, all from the inside. God forbid if you are a physician or anyone else who is too critical and asks too many questions.

During the Vioxx (now discontinued) drug class-action suit in Australia, Merck emails revealed to what lengths they were prepared to go to "neutralize" and "discredit" physicians who were critical of Vioxx. "We may need to seek them out and destroy them where they live," a Merck employee wrote, according to *The Australian*.[334] I personally lost an honorary academic appointment at the University of New Mexico, Department of Pediatrics because of my adamant stance on the removal of thimerosal from vaccines. The individual who would testify on behalf of keeping thimerosal in vaccines at the New Mexico Board of Pharmacy hearings was one of the CDC plants who held an endowed faculty position at UNM. She helped make sure you toed the company line or were removed.

## DON'T BLAME THE DRUG REPS

We like to make fun of drug reps with their blond hair and short, tight dresses bringing meals to physicians and unduly influencing physician-prescribing practices. They are not the problem any more than a small-time drug dealer is responsible for the presence of crack cocaine in the hood. But it still begs the question of how we fix a medical system that has such failings and has gone down, or been led down, so many dead ends so that a few can profit. Clearly, the profit motive must be eliminated almost entirely from as many places in our healthcare system as is feasible.

We look up in the sky and see them spraying us with aluminum and other toxic nanoparticles, and we do nothing. We drink the high-fructose corn syrup and fluoridated water, chew the gum laced with aspartame, and allow ourselves to get vaccinated with deadly ingredients, some of which are meant only to depopulate the world. In the eyes of these deluded psychopathic and self-appointed demigods, we are worthless bottom-feeders who are held in great contempt because they control so much of the world's resources.

The Corporate (Deep) State, the New World Order, globalists, or whatever you want to call them are out to reduce us into mere ants who will either mindlessly work for them or get stepped on. Just never forget that we will always have our individual free will and choice to dissent.

We can oppose the tyranny or wait to get stepped on—that is the choice. Some of us will get stepped on nevertheless, but don't forget we have the power to change all of this by our decisions. We are not stuck, we are not doomed, and we are not limited. Ever!

The children of the Seventh Generation (1989–2012) are just now starting to become adults. This will be their fight, which is why there has been such a strong effort to poison them and dumb them down. Many sacrificed themselves so their uninjured brothers and sisters will know what they need to do when the time comes. That enough will make it through and will be present when called upon is my hope and my prayer.

We are so much more than we have been taught to believe we are. We hold the true power if we choose to use it. Use it or lose it.

*"To sin by silence when they should protest makes cowards of men."*

—Abraham Lincoln

## ADDENDUM FOR *INCURABLE US*

I was initially trained as a pediatrician because I wanted to help children and protect them—I respect them and they deserve respect because it is not easy being human—this is a very challenging planet. Never in my wildest nightmares did I imagine I would be witness to the sanctioned infanticide and democide that has taken place. There are no words for this level of darkness and cruelty. There are no words for the apathy and disregard of those who knew what was going on and said nothing, and did nothing because they wanted to keep their jobs or just wanted to profit from going along with it all—the willfully blind. This is not just about COVID—this human sacrifice has been going on for many decades (worked out really well for the Aztecs). I have nothing to say to these people—again, there are no words—the silent cowards that they are.

I actually feel sorry for them. They will never know in this life what it feels like to have the hand of the divine touch their hearts and feel the boundless love that I know they would seek, if they only knew it was there. Being deprived of that by their own will is the ultimate loss, and while they will find it one day, somewhere, somehow, because there is no separation, for now it is just pathos all around and all the way down. I weep for them as much as I do for their victims.

# Notes

1   https://www.ncbi.nlm.nih.gov/pmc/articles/PMC4797993/
2   Age-stratified infection fatality rate of COVID-19 in the non-elderly informed from pre-vaccination national seroprevalence studies. https://www.medrxiv.org/content/10.1101/2022.10.11.22280963v1.
3   www.ncbi.nlm.nih.gov/books/NBK349040
4   One notable example of a pre-historic civilization being the 12,000-year-old ruins of Göbekli Tepe https://www.worldhistory.org/article/1580/lost-civilisations-of-anatolia-gobekli-tepe/
5   https://vault.fbi.gov/adolf-hitler
6   The symbol was brought to Germany by archaeologist Heinrich Schliemann, noted for his discovery of Troy in 1871.
7   https://www.youtube.com/watch?v=LHHhzCkK4QY
8   https://apnews.com/article/travis-scott-astroworld-music-festival-deaths-ceded-7d0ea08d71b5ce32d4b8218a3fe
9   https://nypost.com/2022/11/30/balenciaga-bdsm-drama-sparks-child-devil-worship-conspiracy theory/
10  Not every member of Bohemian Grove or every visitor is involved, as the puppets bring the very rich and very powerful in as guests—some of whom are clueless about some of the activities that take place there
11  https://www.dailywire.com/news/9-things-you-need-know-about-george-soros-aaron-bandler
12  Satan is not a sinister fellow with a pointed tail who wears red pajamas, Satan is the inversion of love (fear), the inversion of wisdom, the inversion of truth, and the inversion of reality.
13  As already pointed out, it is actually the body that is sold, not the soul.
14  https://www.un.org/humansecurity/agenda-2030
15  https://www.christianobserver.net/documents/the-flouride-deception.pdf
16  https://www.ncbi.nlm.nih.gov/labs/pmc/articles/PMC7305902/
17  https://www.lifesitenews.com/news/vaccine-researcher-admits-big-mistake-says-spike-protein-is-dangerous-toxin/.
18  https://www.ahajournals.org/doi/10.1161/circ.144.suppl_1.10712.
19  https://nypost.com/2021/09/22/wuhan-scientists-wanted-to-release-coronaviruses-into-bats/.

20   DARPA Awards Moderna Therapeutics A Grant For Up To $25 Million To Develop Messenger RNA Therapeutics https://www.prnewswire.com/news-releases/darpa-awards-moderna-therapeutics-a-grant-for-up-to-25-million-to-develop-messenger-rna-therapeutics-226115821.html

21   Blum, William (2006). Rogue State: A Guide to the World's Only Superpower. Zed Books. pp. 150–151. ISBN 978-1-84277-827-2.
     Michael Parenti, The Sword and the Dollar: Imperialism, Revolution, and the Arms Race, St. Martins Press, 1989, pp.74–81.

22   Wheelis, Mark; Rózsa, Lajos; Dando, Malcolm (2006). Deadly cultures: biological weapons since 1945. Harvard University Press. pp. 27–28. ISBN 978-0-674-01699-6. "How the U.S. Government Exposed Thousands of Americans to Lethal Bacteria to Test Biological Warfare". Democracynow.org. July 13, 2005. Retrieved November 2021. https://www.democracynow.org/2005/7/13/how_the_u_s_government_exposed

23   https://www.sciencedirect.com/topics/pharmacology-toxicology-and-pharmaceutical-science/bacillus-globigii.

24   https://exopolitics.org/insiders-reveal-details-of-nasa-usaf-secret-space-programs/; https://www.history.com/this-day-in-history/kennedy-proposes-joint-mission-to-the-moon

25   https://archive.org/stream/pdfy-WRJ-XO7OMYAKus9K/The%20Confession%20That%20Merck%20Pharma%20Created%20The%20Spread%20Of%20AIDS_djvu.txt

26   https://www.washingtonpost.com/archive/opinions/1992/04/05/did-a-polio-vaccine-experiment-unleash-aids-in-africa/0fb7cac2-0b3a-4ec3-8a78-5f032b639bf9/

27   https://asianhealthtalk.wordpress.com/2009/06/26/in-new-theory-swine-flu-started-in-asia-not-mexico/.

28   http://vaccinepapers.org/wp-content/uploads/Introduction-of-DTP-and-OPV-Among-Infants-in-an-Urban-African-Community-A-Natural-Experiment.pdf (https://www.ncbi.nlm.nih.gov/pmc/articles/PMC5360569/)

29   https://www.centerforhealthsecurity.org/our-work/publications/the-spars-pandemic-2025-2028-a-futuristic-scenario-to-facilitate-medical-countermeasure-communication

30   https://centerforhealthsecurity.org/event201/

31   https://www.nature.com/articles/s41591-020-0965-6.

32   https://www.washingtonpost.com/world/2021/10/19/secret-vaccine-contracts-with-governments-pfizer-took-hard-line-push-profit-report-says; https://www.commondreams.org/news/2021/10/19/exposed-how-pfizer-exploits-secretive-vaccine-contracts-strong-arm-governments

33   https://www.politifact.com/article/2021/nov/01/context-never-going-learn-how-safe-vaccine-unless-/

34   https://townhall.com/tipsheet/scottmorefield/2021/10/26/fda-panel-member-were-never-gonna-learn-about-how-safe-the-vaccine-is-until-we-start-giving-it-n2598090.

35  Kanduc, D.: From Genetics to Epigenetics: Top 4 Aspects for Improved Vaccine Designs. Severe Acute Respiratory Syndrome Coronavirus 2 Vaccines as Paradigmatic Examples. Glob Med Genet., November 2021.https://www.thieme-connect.com/products/ejournals/html/10.1055/s-0041-1739495.

36  https://www.commondreams.org/news/2021/10/19/exposed-how-pfizer-exploits-secretive-vaccine-contracts-strong-arm-governments.

37  https://dailysceptic.org/2021/10/28/new-lancet-study-from-sweden-shows-vaccine-effectiveness-against-infection-dropping-to-zero-and-sharp-decline-against-severe-disease-as-well/

38  https://world-signals.com/news/2021/11/22/very-low-levels-of-vaccination-in-africa-low-levels-of-infection/

39  https://www.riotimesonline.com/brazil-news/modern-day-censorship/in-gibraltar-100-of-adults-are-fully-vaccinated-against-covid-19-and-yet-new-cases-are-exploding/

40  https://www.ons.gov.uk/peoplepopulationandcommunity/birthsdeathsandmarriages/deaths/datasets/deathsbyvaccinationstatusengland

41  https://pubmed.ncbi.nlm.nih.gov/33795896/

42  Forever won't last very long for those who keep getting injected.

43  https://link.springer.com/article/10.1007/s00392-022-02129-5.

44  In this newly revised edition, an additional chapter was added (Chapter Nine), which was regrettably left out of the first edition and which goes into detail on this addiction protocol.

45  Cloth masks were the poster child for waste in medicine during the COVID casedemic. Masking had nothing to do with control of the COVID infection except made it worse and everything to do with control and the threat of punishment from the bio-security state.

46  "Identification of LFA-1 as a Candidate Autoantigen in Treatment-Resistant Lyme Arthritis," *Science* 281 (1998): 703–706, doi: 10.1126/science.281.5377.703; Christina Trollmo et al., "Molecular Mimicry in Lyme Arthritis Demonstrated at the Single Cell Level: LFA-1αL Is a Partial Agonist for Outer Surface Protein A-Reactive T Cells," *Journal of Immunology* 166 (2001): 5276–5291, doi: 10.4049/jimmunol.166.8.5286.

47  B. Sharmam et al., "*Borrelia burgdorferi*, the Causative Agent of Lyme Disease, Forms Drug-Tolerant Persister Cells," American Society for Microbiology's *Antimicrobial Agents and Chemotherapy* (AAC).

48  A. Abbot, "Lyme Disease: Uphill Struggle," *Nature* 439 (2006): 524–525, doi:10.1038/439524a.

49  Judith Miklossy, "Alzheimer's Disease-a Neurospirochetosis. Analysis of the Evidence Following Koch's and Hill's Criteria," *Journal of Neuroinflammation* 8 (2011): 90, doi:10.1186/1742–2094–8–90.

50  AB MacDonald, "Alzheimer's neuroborreliosis with trans-synaptic spread of infection and neurofibrillary tangles derived from intraneuronal spirochetes." Med Hypotheses. 2007;68(4):822–825. Epub 2006 Oct 20.

51  Wills and Barry 1991.

52  Donald W. Light, Joel Lexchin, and Jonathan Darrow, "Institutional Corruption of Pharmaceutical Companies and the Myth of Safe and Effective Drugs," *Journal of Law, Medicine and Ethics* 14 (2013): 590–610.

53  Praharaj, "Seroprevalence of *Borrelia burgdorferi* in North Eastern India," *MJAFI*, 64:1, 2008.

54  Daniel J. Cameron, Lorraine B. Johnson, and Elizabeth L. Maloney, "Evidence Assessments and Guideline Recommendations in Lyme Disease: The Clinical Management of Known Tick Bites, Erythema Migrans Rashes and Persistent Disease," *Expert Review of Anti-infective Therapy*, 12:9 (2008): 1103–1135.

55  Lyme Disease Association, Inc., "Conflicts of Interest in Lyme Disease: Laboratory Testing, Vaccination, and Treatment Guidelines" in the conflict report for the Lyme Disease Association, Inc. (Jackson, New Jersey, 2001). See http://www.lymediseaseassociation.org/images/pdf/ConflictReport.pdf.

56  Mary Beth Pfeiffer, "Lyme, the Ties that Bind," *Poughkeepsie Journal*, May 17, 2013; see http://archive.poughkeepsiejournal.com/interactive/article/20130517/WATCHDOG/305160051/INTERACTIVE-Lyme-ties-bind.

57  For example, in 2011 Burton A. Waisbren, MD, a cofounder of the IDSA, published a book: *Treatment of Chronic Lyme Disease: Fifty-One Case Reports and Essays in Their Regard.*

58  "Attorney General's Investigation Reveals Flawed Lyme Disease Guideline Process, IDSA Agrees To Reassess Guidelines, Install Independent Arbiter," State of Connecticut Office of the Attorney General, May 1, 2008, http://www.ct.gov/ag/cwp/view.asp?a=2795&q=414284.

59  Raphael B. Stricker and Lorraine Johnson, "Lyme Disease: The Next Decade," *Infection and Drug Resistance* 4 (2011): 1–9, doi:10.2147/IDR.S15653.

60  Cameron, Johnson, and Maloney, "Evidence Assessments and Guideline Recommendations in Lyme Disease," 2014.

61  "Plum Island's shadowy past: Once-secret documents reveal lab's mission was germ warfare," *Newsday* 3, 1993.

62  Wei-Gang Qiu et al., "Wide Distribution of a High-Virulence *Borrelia burgdorferi* Clone in Europe and North America," *Emerging Infectious Diseases* 14 (2008): 1097–1104, doi:10.3201/eid1407.070880.

63  Knowing that there is evidence of the emergence of a more virulent strain of Bb gives all the more credibility to the history of this facility, as detailed in the book *Lab 257.* Michael Christopher Carroll, *Lab 257: The Disturbing Story of the Government's Secret Plum Island Germ Laboratory* (New York: William Morrow, 2004).

64  It is regrettable that I cannot recommend doing testing at any national lab chain for either the ELISA or Western blot—it is basically a waste of time.

65  A. Vojdani et al., "Novel Diagnosis of Lyme Disease: Potential for CAM Intervention." *Evidence-Based Complement Alternate Med.* 6:3 (2009): 283–295.

66  See http://www.nutramedix.ec/ns/lyme-protocol.

67  See http://www.lymephotos.com.

68  See http://www.klinghardtacademy.com/Protocols/Klinghardt-Biological-treatment-of-Lyme-disease.html.

69  See http://english.storl.de/publications/books/healing-lyme-disease-naturally.html.

70   See http://www.treatlyme.net/lyme-treatment-guidelines.

71   F. W. Schardt, "Clinical Effects of Fluconazole in Patients with Neuroborreliosis," *European Journal of Medical Research* 9 (2004): 334–336.

72   Gao Yuan et al., "Synergistic Effect of Fluconazole and Doxycycline against *Candida albicans* Biofilms Resulting from Calcium Fluctuation and Down Regulation of Fluconazole-Inducible Efflux Pump Gene Overexpression," *J Med Microbiol* 63 (2014): 956–61, doi: 10.1099/jmm.0.072421–0.

73   See http://www.ncbi.nlm.nih.gov/pmc/articles/PMC3594465/.

74   T. Bjarnsholt et al., "Garlic Blocks Quorum Sensing and Promotes Rapid Clearing of Pulmonary Pseudomonas Aeruginosa Infections," *Microbiology* 151 (2005): 3873–3880.

75   M. V. Alvarez et al., "Oregano Essential Oil-Pectin Edible Films as Anti-quorum Sensing and Food Antimicrobial Agents," *Front Microbiology* 5 (2014): 699, doi: 10.3389/fmicb.2014.00699.

76   J. Feng, P. G. Auwaerter, Y. Zhang, "Drug Combinations against *Borrelia burgdorferi* Persisters In Vitro: Eradication Achieved by Using Daptomycin, Cefoperazone and Doxycycline," *PLoS One* 10:3 (2015): e0117207. doi:10.1371/journal.pone.0117207.

77   J. Feng, et al.: A Drug Combination Screen Identifies Drugs Active against Amoxicillin-Induced Round Bodies of *In Vitro Borrelia burgdorferi* Persisters from an FDA Drug Library. Front. Microbiol., 23 May 2016 | http://dx.doi.org/10.3389/fmicb.2016.00743.

78   K. A. Sayler et al., "Isolation of Tacaribe Virus, a Caribbean Arenavirus, from Host-Seeking *Amblyomma americanum* Ticks in Florida." *PLoS One* 9 (2014): e115769, 10.1371/journal.pone.0115769.

79   A virus in the *Thogotovirus* genus of the *Orthomyxoviridae* family

80   Middelveen et al., "Exploring the Association between Morgellons Disease and Lyme Disease: Identification of *Borrelia burgdorferi* in Morgellons Disease Patients," *BMC Dermatology* 15:1 (2015).

81   "Alzheimer's Disease Fact Sheet," National Institute on Aging, last modified June 9, 2015, http://www.nia.nih.gov/alzheimers/publication/alzheimers-disease-fact-sheet.

82   "About the Health and Retirement Study," Institute for Social Research University of Michigan, 2015, http://hrsonline.isr.umich.edu/index.php.

83   Alzheimer's Association, "Alzheimer's Disease Facts and Figures," *Alzheimers Dement* 10 (2014): e47–e92.

84   Keith N. Fargo et al., "2014 Report on the Milestones for the US National Plan to Address Alzheimer's Disease," *The Journal of the Alzheimer's Association* 10 (2014): S430–S452, doi: http://dx.doi.org/10.1016/j.jalz.2014.08.103.

85   J. Weuve et al., "Deaths in the United States among persons with Alzheimer's disease (2010–2050)," *Alzheimers Dement* 10 (2014): e40–46, doi: 10.1016/j.jalz.2014.01.004. See also: https://www.alz.org/facts/downloads/facts_figures_2015.pdf.

86   J. Miklossy, "Alzheimer's Disease—A Neurospirochetosis. Analysis of the Evidence Following Koch's and Hill's Criteria," *Journal of Neuroinflammation* 8 (2011): 90, doi:10.1186/1742-2094-8-90.

87   *T. pectinovorum, T. amylovorum, T. lecithinolyticum, T. maltophilum, T. medium, T. socranskii.*

88  F. Liu et al., "Minocycline Supplementation for Treatment of Negative Symptoms in Early-Phase Schizophrenia: A Double Blind, Randomized, Controlled Trial," *Schizophr Res* 153 (2014): 169–176, doi: 10.1016/j.schres.2014.01.011.

89  S.T. DeKosky and S. Gandy, "Environmental Exposures and the Risk for Alzheimer Disease: Can We Identify the Smoking Guns?," *JAMA Neurol* 71 (2014): 273–275, doi:10.1001/jamaneurol.2013.6031.

90  J. Holder, "Assessment of the Carcinogenicity of Dicofol (Kelthane (Trade Name)), DDT, DDE, and DDD (TDE)," U.S. Environmental Protection Agency, 1986, 2011.

91  G. Koppen et al. *Environ Int*. 35 (2009):1015–1022.

92  Pedercini,et al., "Application of the Malaria Management Model to the Analysis of Costs. Benefits of DDT versus Non DDT Malaria Control," *PLoS ONE* 6, 2011.

93  http://www.premiumtimesng.com/news/141150-african-countries-adopt-contro-versial-deadly-chemical-ddt-for-malaria-treatment.html.

94  T. S. Saraswathy Subramaniam et al., "Viral Aetiology of Acute Flaccid Paralysis Surveillance Cases, before and after Vaccine Policy Change from Oral Polio Vaccine to Inactivated Polio Vaccine," *Journal of Tropical Medicine* 2014 (2014): doi: http://dx.doi.org/10.1155/2014/814908.

95  Janis Gabliks, "Studies of Biologically Active Agents in Cells and Tissue Cultures," Department of Nutrition and Food Science, Massachusetts Institute of Technology, 1966, http://www.dtic.mil/cgi-bin/GetTRDoc?AD=AD0804387&Location=U2&doc=GetTRDoc.pdf.

96  Janis Gabliks and Leo Friedman, "Effects of insecticides on mammalian cells and virus infections," *Annals of the New York Academy of Sciences* 160 (1969, 2006): 254–271, doi: 10.1111/j.1749–6632.1969.tb15846.x.

97  F. Kamel et al., "Pesticide exposure and amyotrophic lateral sclerosis," *Neurotoxicology* 33 (2012): 457–462.

98  K. Hardell et al., "Concentrations of organohalogen compounds and titres of antibodies to Epstein-Barr virus antigens and the risk for non-Hodgkin lymphoma," *Oncol Rep*. 6, June 21, 2009, 1567–1576.

99  http://www.douglasandlondon.com/areas-of-practice/environmental-toxic-exposure/c-8/c-8-details/.

100  Jon Queally, "Glyphosate, Favored Chemical of Monsanto & Dow, Declared 'Probable' Source of Cancer for Humans," *Common Dreams*, March 23, 2015, http://www.commondreams.org/news/2015/03/23/glyphosate-favored-chemical-monsanto-dow-declared-probable-source-cancer-humans.

101  Robin Mesnage et al., "Major Pesticides Are More Toxic to Human Cells Than Their Declared Active Principles" *BioMed Research International* 2014 (2014):179691, doi:10.1155/2014/179691.

102  R. Mesnage, B. Bernay, and G.E. Séralini, "Ethoxylated adjuvants of glyphosate-based herbicides are active principles of human cell toxicity," *Toxicology* 313 (2013):122–128, doi: 10.1016/j.tox.2012.09.006.

103  G.E. Séralini et al., "Answers to critics: why there is a long term toxicity due to Roundup-tolerant genetically modified maize and to a Roundup herbicide," *Food and Chemical Toxicology* 53 (2013):461–468, doi: 10.1016/j.fct.2012.11.007; see also

L.P. Walsh et al., "Roundup inhibits steroidogenesis by disrupting steroidogenic acute regulatory (StAR) protein expression," *Environmental Health Perspectives* 108 (2000):769–776.

104 R. Mesnage et al., "Major Pesticides Are More Toxic to Human Cells Than Their Declared Active Principles." *Biomed Res Int.* 2014: 179691.

105 European Environment Agency, "Late lessons from early warnings: science, precaution, innovation," in the EEA Report (Luxembourg: European Union, 2013), http://www.eea.europa.eu/publications/late-lessons-2.

106 The ADI measure is an assumption based on current understandings of what toxicity might be from long-term exposure to repeated ingestion of chemical compounds in foods (present and/or added), as opposed to acute toxicity. It is a projection often based on skewed if not truncated or biased research. In the case of glyphosate there is an ADI but glyphosate is applied with untested co-forumulants that significantly enhance the synergistic toxicities. It makes the ADI for glyphosate itself misleading even if it were accurate.

107 N. Defarge, et al.: "Co-Formulants in Glyphosate-Based Herbicides Disrupt Aromatase Activity in Human Cells below Toxic Levels." *Int. J. Environ. Res. Public Health* 2016, *13*(3), 264; doi:10.3390/ijerph13030264

108 N. Swanson et al., "Genetically engineered crops, glyphosate and the deterioration of health in the United States of America," *Journal of Organic Systems* 9 (2014): 6–37.

109 Mark Bittman, "Stop Making Us Guinea Pigs," *New York Times*, March 25, 2015, http://www.nytimes.com/2015/03/25/opinion/stop-making-us-guinea-pigs.html?action=click&contentCollection=Music&module=MostEmailed&version=Full&region=Marginalia&src=me&pgtype=article&_r=2.

110 *Elvis Mirzaie et al. v. Monsanto Company*, No. 2:15-CV04361, N.A., Cal. (June 9, 2015).

111 M. Caiati, et al., "PrPC Controls via Protein Kinase A the Direction of Synaptic Plasticity in the Immature Hippocampus," *Journal of Neuroscience*, 33 (2013): 2973–2983, doi:10.1523/JNEUROSCI.4149–12.2013.

112 J.M. Purdey "Ecosystems supporting clusters of sporadic TSEs demonstrate excesses of the radical-generating divalent cation manganese and deficiencies of antioxidant co factors Cu, Se, Fe, Zn," *Medical Hypotheses* 54 (2000): 278–306.

113 Project TENDR: Targeting Environmental Neuro-Developmental Risks. The TENDR Consensus Statement. http://ehp.niehs.nih.gov/EHP358/.

114 http://consumersresearch.org/more-than-5300-water-systems-nationwide-fail-epa-lead-test/.

115 Carey Gillam, "Pesticides in your food? Don't worry, says USDA," *St. Louis Post-Dispatch*, December 19, 2014, http://www.stltoday.com/business/local/pesticides-in-your-food-don-t-worry-says-usda/article_934aebbd-ccc7–509a-86b1–9fca959c-fac2.html.

116 ibid (ref 34).

117 Sarah Lazare, "Suppressing Science for Monsanto? Gorups Demand Investigation of USDA," *Common Dreams*, May 5, 2015, http://www.commondreams.org/news/2015/05/05/suppressing-science-monsanto-groups-demand-investigation-usda.

118 Sebastian Stehle and Ralf Schulz, "Agricultural insecticides threaten surface waters at the global scale," *Proceedings of the National Academy of Sciences* 112 (2015): 5750–5755, doi: 10.1073/pnas.1500232112.

119 See http://www.ncbi.nlm.nih.gov/pmc/articles/PMC1473032.

120 "Maternal residence near agricultural pesticide applications and autism spectrum disorders among children in the California Central Valley," *Environ Health Perspect.* 115 (October 2007): 1482–1499, http://www.ncbi.nlm.nih.gov/pubmed/17938740.

121 Barbara A. Cohn et al., "DDT Exposure in Utero and Breast Cancer" *J Clin Endocrinol Metab.* June 16, 2015, jc20151841, www.ncbi.nlm.nih.gov/pubmed/26079774.

122 https://www.sciencedaily.com/releases/2016/06/160624150813.htm.

123 M.A. Johansson, et al. "Zika and the Risk of Micorcephaly." *N Engl J Med.* 2016 May 25.

124 The following comes from the Oxitec website: "The pest control gene produces a protein called tTAV (tetracycline repressible activator variant), which is able to act as a switch to control the activity of other genes. It's a variant because this gene has been optimised to only work in insect cells. In the modified insects, when the tTAV gene is expressed, the non toxic protein ties up the cell's machinery so its other genes aren't expressed and the insect dies."

These people clearly did not watch *Jurassic Park*! The gene has been modified to only work in insect cells, but something always goes wrong—always!

The modified male mosquito fertilizes a normal female in the wild with the gene to disable her offspring so they don't reach maturity. The mosquitoes were released in Brazil in July of 2015, but did the synthetic gene attach to the DNA of the Zika virus? In the article "Zika virus in Brazil may be mutated strain," the Harvard School of Public Health speculates, as have others, that it has mutated. Did the tTav protein latch on to the virus, and then mess with reproducing humans if a mosquito bites them?

The antibiotic tetracycline is the off switch for this gene, and I suppose pregnant women could take this antibiotic in case they were infected while pregnant, but tetracycline is a Category D drug and not to be given to pregnant women because there is up to a 5 percent chance of birth defects—a real quandary.

125 "The Nobel Prize in Physiology or Medicine 2005," Nobel Media, http://www.nobelprize.org/nobel_prizes/medicine/laureates/2005/illpres/.

126 Douglas Adams, *The Hitchhiker's Guide to the Galaxy* (New York: Del Rey, 1979).

127 Crichton, Michael, "Aliens Cause Global Warming," 17 January 2003 speech at the California Institute of Technology (http://s8int.com/crichton.html or http://online.wsj.com/news/articles/SB122603134258207975 or http://stephenschneider.stanford.edu/Publications/PDF_Papers/Crichton2003.pdf).

128 K.J. Dabos et al., "The effect of mastic gum on Helicobacter pylori: a randomized pilot study," *Phytomedicine* 17 (2010):296–299, doi: 10.1016/j.phymed.2009.09.010.

129 John Stauber and Sheldon Rampton, *Toxic Sludge Is Good for You: Lies, Damn Lies and the Public Relations Industry* (Monroe, ME: Common Courage Press, 2002).

130 ALS Association, "ALS in the Military: Unexpected Consequences of Military Service," ALS Association, February 2013, http://www.alsa.org/assets/pdfs/advocacy/als_military_paper.pdf.

131 Li et al., "Human endogenous retrovirus-K contributes to motor neuron disease," *Science Translational Medicine* 30, Sep 2015:Vol. 7, Issue 307, pp. 307ra153.

132 Genervon Biopharmaceuticals press release Genervon-GM604-Reduced-TDP-43-Protein-Aggregates-Slowed (September 22, 2015).

133 Freya Kamel et al., "Pesticide exposure and amyotrophic lateral sclerosis," *Neurotoxicology* 33 (2012): 457–462, doi:10.1016/j.neuro.2012.04.001.

134 Lewy bodies are a collection eosinophilic inclusions often with misfolded α-synuclein fibrils.

135 G.D. Mellick, "CYP450, genetics and Parkinson's disease: gene × environment interactions hold the key," *Journal of Neural Transmission* 70 (2006):159–165.

136 J. Choi et al., "Oxidative Modifications and Aggregation of Cu,Zn-Superoxide Dismutase Associated with Alzheimer and Parkinson Diseases," *Journal of Biological Chemistry* 280 (2005): 11648–11655.

137 V.N. Uversky et al., "Synergistic effects of pesticides and metals on the fibrillation of alpha-synuclein: implications for Parkinson's disease," *Neurotoxicology* 23 (2002): 527–536.

138 Vladimir N. Uversky, Jie Li, and Anthony L. Fink, "Pesticides directly accelerate the rate of K-synuclein fibril formation: a possible factor in Parkinson's disease," *FEBS Letters* 500 (2001): 105–108, doi:10.1016/S0014–5793(01)02597–2.

139 Thomas Taetzsch and Michelle L. Block, "Pesticides, microglial NOX2, and Parkinson's disease," *Journal of Biochemical and Molecular Toxicology* 27 (2013): 137–149, doi: 10.1002/jbt.21464.

140 Gin-Le He et al., "The amelioration of phagocytic ability in microglial cells by curcumin through the inhibition of EMF-induced pro-inflammatory responses," *Journal of Neuroinflammation* 11 (2014). And Marcus Karlstetter et al., "Curcumin is a potent modulator of microglial gene expression and migration," *Journal of Neuroinflammation* 8 (2011).

141 http://newsroom.ucla.edu/releases/ucla-study-finds-vitamin-d-may-94903.

142 Such as *M. fermentans, M. penetrans, M. pneumoniae, M. genitalium, M. pirum,* and *M. hominis.*

143 Such as doxycycline, ciprofloxacin, azithromycin, clarithromycin, or minocycline in pulsed six-week courses.

144 G. L. Nicolson et al., "Diagnosis and treatment of chronic mycoplasmal infections in Fibromyalgia Syndrome and Chronic Fatigue Syndrome: relationship to Gulf War Illness," *Biomed. Therapy* 16 (1998): 266–271.

145 Barbara C. Tilly et al., "Minocycline in Rheumatoid Arthritis: a 48-week, Double-Blind, Placebo-Controlled Trial," *Annals of Internal Medicine* 122 (1995): 81–89, doi:10.7326/0003–4819–122–2–199501150–00001. And J. R. O'Dell et al., "Treatment of Early Seropositive Rheumatoid Arthritis with Minocycline: Four-year Followup of a Double-blind, Placebo-controlled Trial," *Arthritis and Rheumatology* 42 (1999): 1691–1695.

146 Chensheng Lu, Kenneth M. Warchol, and Richard A. Callahan, "*In situ* replication of honey bee colony collapse disorder," *Bulletin of Insectology* 65 (2012): 99–106.

147 Chensheng Lu, Kenneth M. Warchol, and Richard A. Callahan, "Sub-lethal exposure to neonicotinoids impaired honey bees winterization before proceeding to colony
collapse disorder," *Bulletin of Insectology* 67 (2014): 125–130.

148 A class of neuro-active insecticides chemically similar to nicotine.

149 Chuck Raasch, "Monsanto's Roundup blamed for the decline of the monarch butterfly," *St. Louis Post-Dispatch*, February 4, 2015, http://www.stltoday.com/news/
local/illinois/new-environmental-group-report-attacks-monsanto-s-Roundup-for-
monarch/article_c39ae2ae-679d-59f2-8fd3-a91838376acd.html.

150 Jason R. Richardson et al., "Developmental pesticide exposure reproduces features
of attention deficit hyperactivity disorder," *FASEB Journal* (2015): doi:10.1096/
fj.14–260901fj.14–260901.

151 Christopher Exley, Ellen Rotheray, and David Goulson, "Bumblebee Pupae Contain
High Levels of Aluminium," *PLoS One* 10 (2015): doi: 10.1371/journal.pone.0127665.

152 F. Nafar, K. M. Mearow, "Coconut oil attenuates the effects of amyloid-$\beta$ on cortical
neurons in vitro," *Journal of Alzheimer's Disease* 39 (2014): 233–7, doi: 10.3233/
JAD-131436.

153 P. Wlaz et al., "Anticon- 297 vulsant profile of caprylic acid, a main constituent of the
298 medium-chain triglyceride (MCT) ketogenic diet, in mice," *Neuropharmacology*
62 (2012): 1882–1889.

154 The book *The Ketogenic Diet: A Treatment for Epilepsy* was published in the year
2000, and most of it can be read online. John M. Freeman, Jennifer B. Freeman, and
Millicent T. Kelly, *The Ketogenic Diet: A Treatment for Epilepsy* (New York: Demos
Medical Publishing, 2000).

155 Ingredients to Die For, 2014, http://www.ingredientstodiefor.com.

156 I have also treated a patient with Charcot-Marie Tooth disease and their muscle
strength improved ~30%.

157 "Tuberculosis drug PAS may cure Parkinsons's-like illness," *Journal of Occupational and Environmental Medicine* (2006): 15–37.

158 Most physicians who treat HIV patients know about MAC (*M. avium complex*). The
organism that causes bowel disease is *Mycobacterium avium* subspecies *paratuberculosis* (MAP) and differs genetically from other MAC in having fourteen to eighteen
copies of IS900 and a single cassette of DNA involved in the biosynthesis of surface
carbohydrate. Unlike other MAC, MAP is a specific cause of chronic inflammation
of the intestine in many animal species, including man.

159 RedHill Biopharma Ltd., "RedHill Biopharmaceutical company to Sponsor and
Exhibit Its Ongoing Phase III Crohn's Program at the Israeli IBD Society Meeting,"
GlobeNewswire, Inc., December 2, 2014, http://globenewswire.com/news-relea
se/2014/12/02/687900/10110612/en/RedHill-Biopharmaceutical     company-to-
Sponsor-and-Exhibit-Its-Ongoing-Phase-III-Crohn-s-Program-at-the-Israeli-IBD-
Society-Meeting.html.

160 J. Hermon-Taylor et al., "Causation of Crohn's disease by Mycobacterium avium
subspecies paratuberculosis," *Canadian Journal of Gastroenterology* 14 (2000):
521–539.

161 According to the California Department of Public Health's measles surveillance report,
between December of 2014 and March 2015, there were 132 confirmed measles cases

reported in California residents out of a population of 38.8 million. Forty visited Disneyland, 56% were over the age of twenty. Thirty-four children four and under were affected. No deaths. See also California Department of Public Health, "California Measles Surveillance Update," California Department of Public Health Immunization Branch (Sacramento, California, 2015), http://www.cdph.ca.gov/HealthInfo/discond/Documents/Measles_update_3_-_6_-_2015_public.pdf.

162  L. Storgaard et al., "Survival rate in Crohn's disease and ulcerative colitis," *Scandanavian Journal of Gastroenterology* 14 (1979): 225–230.

163  http://www.activistpost.com/2015/07/alec-behind-recent-push-for-mandatory.html.

164  Marlise Guerrero Schimpf, et al., "Neonatal exposure to a glyphosate based herbicide alters the development of the rat uterus." *Toxicology* (2016) http://dx.doi.org/10.1016/j.tox.2016.06.004.

165  J. M. Armfield and A. J. Spencer, "Consumption of nonpublic water: implications for children's caries experience," *Community Dentistry & Oral Epidemiology* 32 (2004): 283–296.

166  M. Diesendorf et al., "New Evidence on Fluoridation," *Australian and New Zealand Journal of Public Health* 21 (1997): 187–190.

167  F. Wang, et al. "Hyperbaric oxygen therapy for the treatment of traumatic brain injury: a meta-analysis." *Neurol Sci.* 2016 Jan 8. PubMed PMID: 26746238.

168  Vance Trimble, *The Hyperbaric Oxygen, the Uncertain Miracle: The Little-Known Maverick Medical Treatment Which Has Saved the Lives of Thousands of People* (Garden City, NY: Doubleday, 1974), 83–84.

169  Hearing Before the House Labor Health, Education and Welfare Committee, House of Representatives, Labor-HEW Public Witness Testimony, 88th Cong. 1 (1963) (Statement of Hitchock).

170  K.P. Stoller, "Quantification of Neurocognitive Changes Before, During, and After Hyperbaric Oxygen Therapy in a Case of Fetal Alcohol Syndrome," *Pediatrics* 116 (2005): e586–e591.

171  P.G. Harch, et al., "Low pressure hyperbaric oxygen therapy and SPECT brain imaging in the treatment of blast-induced chronic traumatic brain injury (post-concussion syndrome) and post traumatic stress disorder: a case report," *Cases Journal* 2 (2009): 6538.

172  K.P. Stoller, "Hyperbaric oxygen therapy (1.5 ATA) in treating sports related TBI/CTE: two case reports," *Medical Gas Research* 1 (2011): 17.

173  Boguslav H. Fischer, Morton Marks, and Theodore Reich, "Hyperbaric-oxygen treatment of multiple sclerosis: a randomized placebo-controlled, double-blind study," *New England Journal of Medicine* 308 (1983): 181–186, 10.1056/NEJM198301273080402.

174  Carole Sénéchal et al., "Hyperbaric Oxygenation Therapy in the Treatment of Cerebral Palsy: A Review and Comparison to Currently Accepted Therapies," *Journal of American Physicians and Surgeons* 12, 2007.

175  "Hyperbaric Oxygen Therapy in Chronic Traumatic Brain Injury or Post-Traumatic Stress Disorder (NBIRR-1)," U.S. National Institutes of Health, last updated March 31, 2015, http://clinicaltrials.gov/ct2/show/NCT01105962.

176 For example: https://www.merck.com/product/usa/pi_circulars/r/remeron/rem-erontablets_pi.pdf.

177 P.W. Andrews et al., "Primum non nocere: an evolutionary analysis of whether antidepressants do more harm than good," *Frontiers in Psychology* 3 (2012): 117, doi: 10.3389/fpsyg.2012.00117.

178 Y. Lucire and C. Crotty, "Antidepressant-induced akathisia-related homicides associated with diminishing mutations in metabolizing genes of the CYP450 family," *Pharmacogenomics and Personalized Medicine* 2011 (2011): 65–81, doi: 10.2147/PGPM.S17445.

179 Pedro L. Delgado et al., "Sequential catecholamine and serotonin depletion in mirtazapine-treated depressed patients," *International Journal of Neuropsychopharmacology* 5 (2002): 63–66, http://dx.doi.org/10.1017/S1461145702002778.

180 https://www.lawyersandsettlements.com/articles/brain_injury/brain-injury-lawsuit-traumatic-17379.html?utm_expid=3607522–13.Y4u1ixZNSt6o8v_5N8VGVA.0&utm_referrer=http%3A%2F%2Fsearch.aol.com%2Faol%2Fsearch%3Fs_qt%3Dsb%26q%3Dnfl%2Bdeceived%2Btbi%26s_it%3Dcustomfirefoxright-ff.

181 D. R. Gutsaeva et al., "Oxygen-induced mitochondrial biogenesis in the rat hippocampus," *Neuroscience* 137 (2006): 493–504.

182 P. Waalkes et al., "Adjunctive HBO treatment of children with cerebral anoxic injury," *Army Medical Department Journal* (2002): 13–21.

183 Two-year costs within the first two years the service member returns home: PTSD, $5,904 to $10,298 depending on whether we count the lives lost to suicide; major depression, $15,461 to $25,757; co-morbid PTSD and major depression, $12,427 to $16,884. One year costs for traumatic brain injury diagnosis: $25,572 to $30,730 in 2005 for mild cases ($27,259 to $32,759 in 2007 dollars), and $252,251 to $383,221 for moderate or severe cases ($268,902 to $408,519 in 2007 dollars). These costs, largely treating symptoms, continue to have out year costs and out year consequences in terms of disability payments, inability to work, etc. The HBOT *one time* cost for service members who need all 80 treatments averages $16,000 at Medicare Reimbursement rates for a one-hour treatment. HBOT alone, and even HBOT in conjunction with other treatments, is very cost effective. If provided acutely within hours of injury, the treatment is even more effective and massively more cost effective. See Terri Tanielian and Lisa Jaycox, eds., *Invisible Wounds of War: Psychological and Cognitive Injuries, Consequences, and Services to Assist Recovery* (Santa Monica, CA: RAND Corporation, 2008), xxii–xxiii.

184 Alberto Ascherio and Kassandra L. Munger, "Environmental risk factors for multiple sclerosis. Part I: the role of infection," *Annals of Neurology* 61 (2007): 288–99, doi:10.1002/ana.21117.

185 Michael P. Pender and Scott R. Burrows, "Epstein–Barr virus and multiple sclerosis: potential opportunities for immunotherapy," *Clinical & Translational Immunology* 3 (2014): doi:10.1038/cti.2014.25.

186 Tesifón Parrón et al., "Association between environmental exposure to pesticides and neurodegenerative diseases," *Toxicology and Applied Pharmacology* 256 (2011): 379–385, doi:10.1016/j.taap.2011.05.006.

187 http://www.medpagetoday.com/resource-center/multiple-sclerosis/retroviruses/a/44119.

188 Bjørn Andersen Nexø et al., "Treatment of HIV and risk of multiple sclerosis," *Epidemiology* 24 (2013): 331–332, doi: 10.1097/EDE.0b013e318281e48a.

189 Ibid.

190 Carolyn A. Wilson, "Viral Safety Studies in Xenotransplantation and Gene Therapy Products," U.S. Food and Drug Administration, last modified February 12, 2015, http://www.fda.gov/BiologicsBloodVaccines/ScienceResearch/BiologicsResearchAreas/ucm127154.htm.

191 Takayuki Miyazawa, "Endogenous retroviruses as potential hazards for vaccines," *Biologicals* 38 (2010): 371–376, doi:10.1016/j. biologicals.2010.03.003. Also Rokusuke Yoshikawa et al., "Contamination of live attenuated vaccines with an infectious feline endogenous retrovirus (RD-114 virus)," *Archives of Virology* 159 (2014): 399–404, doi: 10.1007/s00705–013–1809–1.

192 Irena Milicevic et al., "Ribavirin reduces clinical signs and pathological changes of experimental autoimmune encephalomyelitis in Dark Agouti rats," *Journal of Nueroscience Research* 72 (2003): 268–278, doi: 10.1002/jnr.10552.

193 Kari K. Nissen et al., "Endogenous retroviruses and multiple sclerosis–new pieces to the puzzle," *BMC Neurology* 13 (2013): doi: 10.1186/1471–2377–12–111.

194 Hilary D. Wilson et al., "Hyperbaric Oxygen Treatment Is Comparable to Acetylsalicylic Acid Treatment in an Animal Model of Arthritis," *Journal of Pain* 8 (2007): 924–930, doi:10.1016/j.jpain.2007.06.005.

195 T. Kamada, "Superoxide dismutase and hyperbaric oxygen therapy of the patient with rheumatoid arthritis," *Nihon Seikeigeka Gakkai Zasshi* 59 (1985): 17–26.

196 Philippe Grandjean, Katherine T. Herz, "Methylmercury and brain development: imprecision and underestimation of developmental neurotoxicity in humans," *Mount Sinai Journal of Medicine* 78 (2011): 107–118; Donna Mergler et al., "Methylmercury exposure and health effects in humans: a worldwide concern," *Ambio* 36 (2007): 3–11, doi: 10.3390/ijerph7062666.

197 Joseph L. Jacobson et al., "Relation of Prenatal Methylmercury Exposure from Environmental Sources to Childhood IQ," *Environmental Health Perspectives*: doi:10.1289/ehp.1408554.

198 Christopher A. Shaw et al., "Aluminum-Induced Entropy in Biological Systems: Implications for Neurological Disease," *Journal of Toxicology* 2014: doi:http://dx.doi.org/10.1155/2014/491316.

199 https://www.cia.gov/news-information/speeches-testimony/2016-speeches-testimony/director-brennan-speaks-at-the-council-on-foreign-relations.html.

200 "Field Campaigns," ARM Climate Facility Research, http://www.arm.gov/campaigns/table.

201 Raymond Wiley and KT Prime, *The Georgia Guidestones: America's Most Mysterious Monument* (Hartwell, GA: Elberton Granite Finishing Co., 1981).

202 Steven Watson, "UN Climate Change Official Says 'We Should Make Every Effort' To Depopulate the Planet," *RedFlag News,* April 6, 2015, http://www.redflagnews.com/headlines-2015/video-un-climate-change-official-says-we-should-make-every-effort-to-depopulate-the-planet.

203  Lucio G. Costa et al., "Developmental neuropathology of environmental agents," *Annual Review of Pharmacology and Toxicology* 44 (2004): 87–110, doi: 10.1146/annurev.pharmtox.44.101802.121424. Also Philip W. Davidson, Gary J. Myers, and Bernard Weiss, "Mercury exposure and child development outcomes," *Pediatrics* 113 (2004):1023–1029.

204  Janet Raloff, "Mercurial Risks from Acid's Reign," *New Scientist* 139 (1991): 152–156; Michael Cross, "Review: Minamata and the Search for Justice," *New Scientist* 1756 (1991). And W. Eugene Smith and Aileen M. Smith, *Minamata: The Story of the Poisoning of a City, and of the People Who Chose to Carry the Burden of Courage* (New York: Holt, Rinehart, and Winston, 1975).

205  S. Bernard et al., "Autism: a novel form of mercury poisoning," *Medical Hypotheses* 56 (2001): 462–471, doi:10.1054/mehy.2000.1281. And S. Bernard et al., "The role of mercury in the pathogenesis of autism," *Molecular Psychiatry* 7 (2002): mS42–mS43; Mark F. Blaxill, "Study fails to establish diagnostic substitution as a factor in increased rate of autism," *Pharmacotherapy* 24 (2004): 812–813, doi: 10.1592/phco.24.8.812.36060; Mark F. Blaxill, "What's going on? The question of time trends in autism," *Public Health Reports* 119 (2004): 536–551.

206  Joachim Mutter et al., "Amalgam risk assessment with coverage of references up to 2005," *Gesundheitswesen* 67 (2005):204–216.

207  Mark F. Blaxill, Lyn Redwood, and Sallie Bernard, "Thimerosal and autism? A plausible hypothesis that should not be dismissed," *Medical Hypotheses* 62 (2004): 788–794, doi: http://dx.doi.org/10.1016/j.mehy.2003.11.033.

208  1982, vol. 47, No. 2, *Federal Register*.

209  Centers for Disease Control and Prevention, "Thimerosal in Vaccines: A Joint Statement of the American Academy of Pediatrics and the Public Health Service," *Morbidity and Mortality Weekly Report*, July 9, 1999, http://www.cdc.gov/mmwr/preview/mmwrhtml/mm4826a3.htm.

210  Leslie K. Ball, Robert Ball, and R. Douglas Pratt, "An Assessment of Thimerosal Use in Childhood Vaccines," *Pediatrics* 107 (2001): 1147–1154, doi: 10.1542/peds.107.5.1147.

211  G. V. Stajich et al., "Iatrogenic Exposure to Mercury after Hepatitis B Vaccination in Preterm Infants," *The Journal of Pediatrics* May 2000, 136(5): 79–81

212  Thomas Verstraeten, Robert Davis, and Frank DeStefano, "Thimerosal VSD Study, Phase I," February 29, 2000.

213  Michael E. Pichichero et al., "Mercury concentrations and metabolism in infants receiving vaccines containing thiomersal: a descriptive study," *Lancet* 360 (2002): 1737–1741, doi:10.1016/S0140–6736(02)11682–5.

214  "Simpsonwood Meeting on Mercury and Puerto Rico Meeting on Aluminum," retreat transcript, 2000.

215  Thomas Verstraeten et al., "Vaccine Safety Datalink Team: Safety of thimerosal containing vaccines: a two phased study of computerized health maintenance organization databases," *Pediatrics* 112 (2003): 1039–1048.

216  William W. Thompson, "Statement of William W. Thompson, Ph.D., Regarding the 2004 Article Examining the Possibility of a Relationship Between MMR Vaccine and Autism," Morgan Verkamp LLC, August 27, 2014, http://www.morganverkamp.

com/august-27–2014-press-release-statement-of-william-w-thompson-ph-d-regarding-the-2004-article-examining-the-possibility-of-a-relationship-between-mmr-vaccine-and-autism/.

217 "CDC Whistleblower: Mercury in Vaccines Given to Pregnant Women Linked to Autism," *Health Impact News*, August 27, 2014, http://healthimpactnews.com/2014/cdc-whistle-blower-mercury-in-vaccines-given-to-pregnant-women-causes-autism/.

218 See https://oig.hhs.gov/fraud/fugitives/profiles.asp.

219 See https://oig.hhs.gov/fraud/fugitives/profiles.asp.

220 See http://www.ncbi.nlm.nih.gov/pubmed/23404041.

221 The transcripts of the IOM meetings are available online at www.nomercury.org/iom.htm.

222 Immunization Safety Review Committee, *Immunity Safety Review: Thimerosal-Containing Vaccines and Neurodevelopmental Disorders* (Washington, DC: National Academies Press, 2001).

223 adverse neurodevelopmental disorders

224 David A. Geier and Mark R. Geier, "Early downward trends in neurodevelopmental disorders following removal of Thimerosal-containing vaccines," *Journal of American Physicians and Surgeons*, 11 (2006): 8–13.

225 Jeff Bradstreet, "A case control study of mercury burden in children with autistic disorders and measles virus genomic RNA in cerebrospinal fluid in children with regressive autism" in *Immunization Safety Review: Vaccines and Autism*, Immunization Safety Review Committee (Washington, DC: National Academies Press, 2004).

226 "Mass Sterilization: Kenyan Doctors Find Anti-Fertility Agent in UN Tetanus Vaccine," November 8, 2014, by Steve Weatherbe, www.earth-heal.com.

227 https://www.lifesitenews.com/news/kenyan-bishops-still-wary-despite-new-tests-showing-no-sterilizing-agent-in.

228 Ibid.

229 Peter Ndumbe and Emmanuel Yenshu, "Cameroon: Vaccination and Politics," *Lancet* 339 (May 16, 1992): 1222.

230 Zeitschrift fuer angewandte Chemie, 29. Jahrgang, 15. April 1926, Nr. 15, S. 461–466, Die *Gefaehrlichkeit des Quecksilberdampfes*, von Alfred Stock (1926) http://web.stanford.edu/~bcalhoun/AStock.htm.

231 N.D. Boyd et al., "Mercury from dental 'silver' tooth fillings impairs sheep kidney function," *American Journal of Physiology* 261 (1991): R1010–R1014.

232 Wael Mortada et al., "Mercury in dental restoration: Is there a risk of nephrotoxicity?" *Journal of Nephrology* 15 (2002): 171–176.

233 Sabrina Cedrola et al., "Inorganic mercury changes the fate of murine CNS stem cells," *FASEB Journal* 17 (2003): 869–871, doi:10.1096/fj.02–0491fje. Also Christopher C. W. Leong, Naweed I. Syed, Fritz L. Lorscheider, "Retrograde degeneration of neurite membrane structural integrity of nerve growth cones following in vitro exposure to mercury," *Neuroreport* 12 (2001): 733–737.

234 Edward F. Duhr et al., "HgEDTA Complex Inhibits GTP Interactions with the E-site of Brain betatubulin," *Toxicology and Applied Pharmacology* 122 (1993): 273–280. Also J.T. Ely, "Mercury induced Alzheimer's disease: accelerating incidence?" *Bulletin of Environmental Contamination and Toxicolology* 67 (2001): 800–806;

J. Mutter et al., "Amalgam studies: Disregarding basic principles of mercury toxicity," *International Journal of Hygiene and Environmental Health* 207 (2004): 391–397, doi:10.1078/1438–4639–00305; G. Olivieri et al., "Mercury induces cell cytotoxicity and oxidative stress and increases β-amyloid secretion and τ-phosphorylation in SHSY5Y neuroblastoma cells," *Journal Neurochemistry* 74 (2000): 231–236; G. Olivieri et al., "The effects of betaestradiol on SHSY5Y neuroblastoma cells during heavy metal induced oxidative stress, neurotoxicity and betaamyloid secretion," *Neuroscience* 113 (2002): 849–855, doi: 10.1016/S0306–4522(02)00211–7; James C. Pendergrass et al., "Mercury vapor inhalation inhibits binding of GTP to tubulin in rat brain: similarity to a molecular lesion in Alzheimer diseased brain," *NeuroToxicology* 18 (1997): 315–324.

235 Karolin Ask et al., "Inorganic mercury and methyl mercury in placentas of Swedish women," *Environmental Health Perspectives* 110 (2002): 523–526. See also G. Drasch et al., "Mercury burden of human fetal and infant tissues," *European Journal of Pediatrics* 153 (1994): 607–610.

236 Amy S. Holmes, Mark F. Blaxill, and Boyd E. Haley, "Reduced levels of mercury in first baby haircuts of autistic children," *International Journal of Toxicology* 22 (2003): 277–285, doi: 10.1080/10915810390220054.

237 P. Grandjean, Pal Weihe, and R.F. White, "Milestone development in infants exposed to methylmercury from human milk," *Neurotoxicology* 16 (1995): 27–33.

238 Diana Echeverria et al., "Neurobehavioral effects from exposure to dental amalgam Hg(o): New distinctions between recent exposure and Hg body burden," *FASEB Journal* 12 (1998): 971–980. Also by Robert L. Siblerud, "The relationship between mercury from dental amalgam and mental health," *American Journal of Psychotherapy* 43 (1989): 575–587 and "A comparison of mental health of multiple sclerosis patients with silver/mercury dental fillings and those with fillings removed," *Psychological Reports* 70 (1992): 1139–1151. See also the following two articles by Robert L. Siblerud, Eldon Kienholz, and John Motl: "Evidence that mercury from silver dental fillings may be an etiological factor in smoking," *Toxicology Letters* 68 (1993): 307–310, doi: 10.1016/0378–4274(93)90022-P; "Psychometric evidence that mercury from silver dental fillings maybe an etiological factor in depression, excessive anger, and anxiety," *Psychological Reports* 74 (1994): 67–80.

239 Jarina Bártová et al., "Dental amalgam as one of the risk factors in autoimmune diseases," *Neuroendocrinology Letters* 24 (2003): 65–67; Per Hultman et al., "Adverse immunological effects and autoimmunity induced by dental amalgam and alloy in mice," *FASEB Journal* 8 (1994): 1183–1190; Per Hultman, U. Lindh, and P. Horsted-Bindslev, "Activation of the immune system and systemic immune complex Amalgam studies 395 deposits in Brown Norway rats with dental amalgam restorations," *Journal of Dental Research* 77 (1998): 1415–1425; Jarmila Prochazkova et al., "The beneficial effects of amalgam replacement on health of patients with autoimmunity," *Neuroendocrinology Letters* 25 (2004): 211–218; J. Stejskal and Vera D. Stejskal, "The role of metals in autoimmunity and the link to neuroendocrinology," *Neuroendocrinology Letters* 20 (1999): 351–364; Ivan Sterzl et al., "Mercury and nickel allergy: Risk factors in fatigue and autoimmunity," *Neuroendocrinology Letters* 20 (1999): 221–228; C.S. Via et al., "Low dose exposure to inorganic mercury

accelerates disease and mortality in acquired murine lupus," *Environmental Health Perspectives* 111 (2003): 1273–1277.

240 Lin-Wen Hu, John A. Bernard, and Jianmei Che, "Neutron activation analysis of hair samples for the identification of autism," *Transactions of the American Nuclear Society* 89 (2003): 681–682.

241 Personal communication with the retired chairman of the chemistry department of the University of Kentucky, Boyd Haley.

242 Maths Berlin, "Mercury in dental filling materials—an updated risk analysis in environmental medical terms," The Dental Material Commission Care and Consideration, 2003, http://www.drfarid.com/Swedish%20mercury.pdf.

243 Institute for Water, Soil and Air Hygiene of the Federal Environment Agency, "Monograph on mercury—reference and human biomonitoring values (HBM)," *Health Research* 42 (1999): 522–532.

244 G. Mark Richardson, "Assessment of Mercury Exposure and Risks from Dental Amalgam," final report, Medical Devices Bureau (Ottawa, CA, 1995), http://mercurypoisoned.com/research/mark_richardson_final_report.pdf.

245 William E. Brooks et al., U.S. Department of the Interior, U.S. Geological Survey, "Peru Mercury Inventory 2006," open-file report 2007–1252, U.S. Geological Survey (Reston, Virginia, 2006), http://pubs.usgs.gov/of/2007/1252/ofr2007–1252.pdf.

246 Truth Revealed: New Scientific Discoveries Regarding Mercury in Medicine and Autism: Hearing Before the Subcommittee on Human Rights and Wellness, House of Representatives, 108th Cong. 2 (2004) (Statement of Richard C. Deth, Bouve College of Health Sciences, Department of Pharmaceutical Services, Northeastern University).

247 Josef Warkany and Donald M. Hubbard, "Acrodynia and mercury," *Journal of Pediatrics* 42 (1953): 365–386, doi:http://dx.doi.org/10.1016/S0022–3476(53)80195–2.

248 Dave Weldon, "Immunization Safety Review: Vaccines and Autism," presented at public meeting for Institute of Medicine, Washington, DC, February 9, 2004. See also Lyn Redwood, Truth Revealed: New Scientific Discoveries Regarding Mercury in Medicine and Autism: Hearing Before the Subcommittee on Human Rights and Wellness, House of Representatives, 108th Cong. 2 (2004) (Statement of Lyn Redwood, president, Coalition for Safeminds); David Willman, "The National Institutes of Health: Public Servant or Private Marketer?," *Los Angeles Times*, December 22, 2004, http://www.latimes.com/news/la-na-nih22dec22-story.html#page=4; Richard Fischer, Truth Revealed: New Scientific Discoveries Regarding Mercury in Medicine and Autism: Hearing Before the Subcommittee on Human Rights and Wellness, House of Representatives, 108th Cong. 2 (2004) (Statement of Richard Fischer, International Academy of Oral Medicine and Toxicology); Mark R. Geier and David A. Geier, "Mercury in vaccines and potential conflicts of interest," *Lancet* 364 (2004): 1217, doi:http://dx.doi.org/10.1016/S0140–6736(04)17133-X.

249 J. Mutter and F. D. Daschner, "Commentary regarding the article by Gottwald et al., 'Amalgam disease'—poisoning, allergy, or psychic disorder?" *International Journal of Hygiene and Environmental Health* 206 (2003): 69–70; H. Walach et al., "No difference between self reportedly amalgam sensitives and nonsensitives?

Listen carefully to the data," *International Journal of Hygiene and Environmental Health* 206 (2003): 139–141.

250  Birgit Gottwald, "Amalgam disease—poisoning, allergy, or psychic disorder?" *International Journal of Hygiene and Environmental Health* 204 (2001): 223–229, doi:10.1078/1438–4639–00097 [translated citation from German]; Birgit Gottwald et al., "Response regarding the critical remarks by Mutter and Daschner," *International Journal of Hygiene and Environmental Health* 206 (2003): 71–73, doi: 10.1078/1438–4639–00186; Life Science Research Office, "Review and Analysis of the Literature on the Health Effects of Dental Amalgams," final report, the Transagency Working Group on the Health Effects of Dental Amalgam U.S. Department of Health and Human Services (Rockville, Maryland, 2004) https://www.faseb.org/Portals/2/PDFs/LSRO_Legacy_Reports/2004_%20Review%20and%20Analysis%20of%20the%20Literature%20on%20the%20Potential%20Adverse%20Haealth%20Effects%20of%20Dental%20Amalgam_REPORT%20SUPPLEMENT%202009–07–2004.pdf; John E. Dodes, "The amalgam controversy: An evidence based analysis," *Journal of the American Dental Association* 132 (2001): 348–356.; *Amalgams in Dental Therapy*, Federal Institute for Pharmaceuticals and Medical Products (Bonn: Federal Institute for Pharmaceuticals and Medical Products, 2005); R. Harhammer, "The risk assessment of the dental filling material amalgam," *Health Research* 44 (2001): 149–154, doi: 10.1007 / s001030050424. See also the following by Holger Zimmer et al., "Determination of mercury in blood, urine and saliva for the biological monitoring of an exposure from amalgam fillings in a group with self reported adverse health effects," *International Journal of Hygiene and Environmental Health* 205 (2002): 205–211, doi:10.1078/1438–4639–00146; "Response to the letter of Walach et al., Int. J. Hyg. Environ. Health, 2003;206:139–41," *International Journal of Hygiene and Environmental Health* 206 (2003): 143–145, doi: 10.1078/1438–4639–00204.

251  http://www.miamiherald.com/news/nation-world/national/article28027159.html.

252  L. Magos et al., "The comparative toxicology of ethyl and methyl mercury," *Archives of Toxicology* 57 (1985): 260–267, doi:10.1007/BF00324789.

253  Thomas M. Burbacher et al., "Comparison of blood and brain mercury levels in infant monkeys exposed to methylmercury or vaccines containing thimerosal," *Environmental Health Perspectives* 113 (2005): 1015–1021, doi: 10.1289/ehp.7712.

254  methylmercury [MeHg] [CASRN 22967–92–6], www.epa.gov/iris/subst/0073.htm.

255  M. Waly et al., "Activation of methionine synthase by insulin-like growth factor1 and dopamine: A target for neurodevelopmental toxins and thimerosal," *Molecular Psychiatry* 9 (2004): 358–370.

256  S. Jill James et al., "Metabolic biomarkers of increased oxidative stress and impaired methylation capacity in children with autism," *American Journal of Clinical Nutrition* 80 (2004): 1611–1617.

257  Jeff Bradstreet et al., "A Case-Control Study of Mercury Burden in Children with Autistic Spectrum Disorders," *Journal of American Physicians and Surgeons* 8 (2003): 76–79.

258 Thomas Stoiber et al., "Disturbed microtubule function and induction of micronuclei by chelate complexes of mercury (II)," *Mutation Research/Genetic Toxicology and Environmental Mutagenesis* 563 (2004): 97–106, doi:10.1016/j.mrgentox.2004.06.009.

259 Joachim Mutter et al., "Alzheimer Disease: Mercury as pathogenetic factor and apolipoprotein E as a moderator," *Neuroendocrinology Letters* 25 (2004): 275–283.

260 David S Baskin, Hop Ngo, and Vladimir V Didenko, "Thimerosal induces DNA breaks, caspase3 activation, membrane damage, and cell death in cultured human neurons and fibroblasts," *Toxicological Sciences* 74 (2003): 361–368.

261 Götz A. Westphal et al., "Thimerosal induces micronuclei in the cytochalasin B block micronucleus test with human lymphocytes," *Archive of Toxicology* 77 (2003): 50–55, doi: 10.1007/s00204–002–0405-z.

262 E. Colmann et al., "Mercury in infants given vaccines containing thimerosal," *Lancet* 361 (2003): 698–699.

263 S. Jill James et al., "Thimerosal neurotoxicity is associated with glutathione depletion: protection with glutathione precursors," *Neurotoxicology* 26 (2005): 18.

264 M. Muller et al., "Inhibition of the human erythrocytic glutathione-S-transferase T1 (GST T1) by thimerosal," *International Journal of Hygiene and Environmental Health* 203 (2001): 479–481.

265 A. Vojdani et al., "Infections, toxic chemicals and dietary peptides binding to lymphocyte receptors and tissue enzymes are major instigators of autoimmunity in autism," *International Journal of Immunopathology Pharmacology* 16 (2003): 189–199.

266 Miguel A. Hernan et al., "Recombinant hepatitis B vaccine and the risk of multiple sclerosis: a prospective study," *Neurology* 63 (2004): 838–842.

267 Diana L. Vargas et al., "Neuroglial activation and neuroinflammation in the brain of patients with autism," *Annals of Neurology* 57 (2005): 67–81.

268 Mady Hornig, D. Chian, and W.I. Lipkin, "Neurotoxic effects of postnatal thimerosal are mouse strain dependent," *Molecular Psychiatry* 9 (2004): 833–845, doi:10.1038/sj.mp.4001529.

   Mady Hornig, Truth Revealed: New Scientific Discoveries Regarding Mercury in Medicine and Autism: Hearing Before the Subcommittee on Human Rights and Wellness, House of Representatives, 108th Cong. 2 (2004) (Statement of Mady Hornig, assistant professor of epidemiology, Columbia University).

269 G.A. Westphal et al., "Homozygous gene deletions of the glutathione Stransferases M1 and T1 are associated with thimerosal sensitization," *International Archive of Occupational and Environmental Health* 73 (2000): 384–388.

270 Boyd Haley, "Reduced levels of mercury in first baby haircuts of Autistic children" (presented at public meeting for Institute of Medicine, Washington, DC, February 9, 2004).

271 Jack Schubert, E. Joan Riley, and Sylvanus A. Tyler, "Combined effects in toxicology—a rapid systematic testing procedure: cadmium, mercury, and lead," *Journal of Toxicology and Environmental Health* 4 (1978): 763–776, doi:10.1080/15287397809529698.

272 Mark R. Geier and David A. Geier, "Neurodevelopmental disorders after thimerosal containing vaccines: A brief communication," *Experimental Biology and Medicine*

228 (2003): 660–664. See also by the same authors: "An assessment of the impact of thimerosal on childhood neurodevelopmental disorders," *Pediatric Rehabilitation* 6 (2003): 97–102, doi: 10.1080/1363849031000139315; "Thimerosal in childhood vaccines, neurodevelopment disorders, and heart disease in the U.S.," *Journal of American Physicians and Surgeons* 8 (2003): 6–11; "A comparative evaluation of the effects of MMR immunization and mercury doses from thimerosal containing childhood vaccines on the population prevalence of autism," *Medical Science Monitor* 10 (2004): PI33–PI39; "Autism and thimerosal containing vaccines: Analysis of the vaccine adverse events reporting system (VAERS)" (presented at public meeting for Institute of Medicine, Washington, DC, February 9, 2004).

273 Kreesten M. Madsen et al., "Thimerosal and the Occurrence of Autism: Negative Ecological Evidence From Danish Population Based Data," *Pediatrics* 112 (2003): 604–606; Anders Hviid et al., "Association Between Thimerosal Containing Vaccine and Autism," *Journal of the American Medical Association* 290 (2003): 1763–1766, doi:10.1001/jama.290.13.1763; Paul Stehr-Green et al., "Autism and Thimerosal-containing vaccines: lack of consistent evidence for an association," *American Journal of Preventive Medicine* 25 (2003),101–106, doi:10.1016/S0749–3797(03)00113–2; Safe Minds, "Analysis of the Danish Autism Registry Database in Response to the Hviid et al Paper on Thimerosal in *JAMA* (October, 2003)," by Sallie Bernard (Cranford, New Jersey), http://www.putchildrenfirst.org/media/5.18.pdf.

274 1982, Vol. 47, No. 2, *Federal Register*.

275 J. P. Leigh and J. Du, "Brief Report: Forecasting the Economic Burden of Autism in 2015 and 2025 in the United States," *J Autism Dev Disord.*, July 17, 2015.

276 Tom Jefferson, "Influenza vaccination: Policy versus evidence," *BMJ* 333 (2006): 912–915, doi: 10.1136/bmj.38995.531701.80; David A. Geier, Paul G. King, and Mark R. Geier, "Influenza Vaccine: Review of effectiveness of the U.S. immunization program, and policy considerations," *Journal of American Physicians and Surgeons* 11 (2006): 69–74.

277 See http://www.fda.gov/cber/vaccine/thimerosal.htm.

278 See http://www.ajph.org/cgi/eletters/AJPH.2007.113159v1; also David Kirby, "Government Concedes Vaccine-Autism Case in Federal Court—Now What?," *Huffington Post*, November 17, 2011, http://www.huffingtonpost.com/david-kirby/government-concedes-vacci_b_88323.html.

279 See Parran et al., *Toxicol Sci* 2005; 86: 132–140.

280 See http://www.epa.gov/safewater/contaminants/index.html#mcls.

281 See Leong et al., *Neuroreport* 2001; 12: 733–737.

282 See http://www.epa.gov/epaoswer/hazwaste /mer cury/ regs.htm#hazwaste.

283 Brian Hooker et al., "Review Article: Methodological Issues and Evidence of Malfeasance in Research Purporting to Show Thimerosal in Vaccines Is Safe," *BioMed Research International* 2014 (2014): doi:10.1155/2014/247218.

284 Dick Carozza, "FDA Incapable of Protecting U.S., Scientist Alleges," *Fraud Magazine*, September/October 2005, http://www.fraud-magazine.com/article.aspx?id=4294967770.

285 Bill Gates, "Innovating to zero!," TED, 27:49, February 2010, http://www.ted.com/talks/bill_gates.

286  Peter Aaby et al., "Differences in female-male mortality after high-titre measles vaccine and association with subsequent vaccination with diphtheria-tetanus-pertussis and inactivated poliovirus: a re-analysis of the West African studies," *Lancet* 361 (2003): 2183–2188, doi:10.1016/S0140–6736(03)13771–3.

287  https://www.washingtonpost.com/news/wonk/wp/2014/09/29/our-infant-mortality-rate-is-a-national-embarrassment/.

288  http://www.cdc.gov/vaccines/vac-gen/howvpd.htm

289  Frank Shann, "The non-specific effects of vaccines," *Archives of Disease in Childhood* 95 (2010): 662–667.

290  Benjamin M. Althouse and Samuel V. Scarpino, "Asymptomatic transmission and the resurgence of Bordetella pertussis," *BMC Medicine* 13(2015): doi: 10.1186/s12916–015–0382–8.

291  Stanley Plotkin, Walter Orsenstein, and Paul Offit, *Vaccines* (Philadelphia: Elsevier; 2008).

292  Jabism is not a real religion; I made it up for this book. Any similarity to a real religion or an imagined religion is purely coincidental.

293  http://www.thenewamerican.com/tech/environment/item/6700-was-swine-flu-outbreak-caused-by-lab-leak.

294  Jon Rappoport, "Globalism and the push for mandatory universal vaccination," *John Rappoport's Blog*, June 11, 2015, https://jonrappoport.wordpress.com/2015/06/11/globalism-and-the-push-for-mandatory-universal-vaccination/.

295  "A Systematic Review of the Evidence on the Effectiveness and Risks of Inactivated Influenza Vaccines in Different Target Groups," *Vaccine* 29 (2011): 9159–9170.

296  http://www.aapsonline.org/testimony/mandvac.htm.

297  "Romark Laboratories Initiates Phase 3 Trial Of New Influenza Drug," Romark Laboratories, L.C., April 18, 2013, http://www.romark.com/news/11-uncategorised/48-romark-laboratories-initiates-phase-3-trial-of-new-influenza-drug.

298  Jae-Min Song, Kwang-Hee Lee, Baik-Lin Seong, "Antiviral effect of catechins in green tea on influenza virus,"*Antiviral Research* 68 (2005): 66–74, doi:10.1016/j.antiviral.2005.06.010; Mikio Nakayama et al., "Inhibition of the infectivity of influenza virus by tea polyphenols," *Antiviral Research* 21 (1993): 289–299, doi:10.1016/0166–3542(93)90008–7; Kunihiro Kaihatsu et al., "Broad and potent anti-influenza virus spectrum of epigallocatechin-3-O-gallate-monopalmitate," *Journal of Molecular and Genetic Medicine* 3 (2009): 195–197.

299  M. Urashima et al., "Randomized trial of vitamin D supplementation to prevent seasonal influenza A in schoolchildren," *American Journal of Clinical Nutrition* 91 (2010): 1255–1260, doi: 10.3945/ajcn.2009.29094.

300  M. Zu et al., "In vitro anti-influenza virus and anti-inflammatory activities of theaflavin derivatives," *Antiviral Research* 94 (2012): 217–224, doi: 10.1016/j.antiviral.2012.04.001.

301  Liang Jin et al., "Indole-3-Carbinol Prevents Cervical Cancer in Human Papilloma Virus Type 16 (HPV16) Transgenic Mice," *Cancer Research* 59 (1999): 3991–3997; Maria C. Bell et al., "Placebo-Controlled Trial of Indole-3-Carbinol in the Treatment of CIN," *Gynecologic Oncology* 78 (2000): 123–129, doi:10.1006/gyno.2000.5847.

302 Eliseeva M. Yu, et al., "Antiviral effect of isoprinosine in HPV-associated diseases," *Obstetrics and Gynecology* 2 (2012).

303 A.G. Kedrova et al., "Role of antiviral therapy in the complex treatment of patients with epithelial dysplasias and preinvasive cancer of the cervix uteri," *Obstetrics and Gynecology* 6 (2006).

304 The newly approved Gardasil vaccine now covers nine strains.

305 FDA's VRBPAC Background document, used at the May 18, 2006 meeting where Gardasil approval was discussed: "Concerns Regarding Primary Endpoint Analyses among Subgroups" (presented at Gardasil HPV Quadrivalent Vaccine VRBPAC meeting for FDA, May 18, 2006): 13. "Study 013: Analysis of efficacy against vaccine-relevant HPV types CIN 2/3 or worse among subjects who were PCR positive and/or seropositive for the relevant HPV type at day 1" (presented at Gardasil HPV Quadrivalent Vaccine VRBPAC meeting for FDA, May 18, 2006): 14, Table 19. Table 19 shows that the efficacy rate for this group to be -33.7% (a negative efficacy number means the vaccine led to an INCREASED risk of disease in the subgroups mentioned). "Detailed Safety Population: Number (%) of subjects who reported systemic adverse reactions of 2% or greater in the 15 days following receipt of study vaccine " (presented at Gardasil HPV Quadrivalent Vaccine VRBPAC meeting for FDA, May 18, 2006):22, Table 32. Table 32 shows that the number of subjects reporting systemic adverse reactions was 3591. That is a percentage of 59.2% of the participants.

306 "H.pylori eradication may shorten life span," *Med Check* 1 (2015): 1–14.

307 http://sanevax.org/wp-content/uploads/2015/11/Gomez-v-USDOH-expert-report.pdf.

308 Ibid.

309 http://www.fas.org/sgp//crs/misc/RS22327.pdf.

310 Scot J. Paltrow, "Behind the Pentagon's doctored ledgers, a running tally of epic waste," *Reuters Investigates*, November 18, 2013, http://www.reuters.com/investigates/pentagon/#article/part2.

311 http://www.thefiscaltimes.com/Articles/2013/11/27/Accounting-Fraud-Defense-Department-Shocking.

312 Fiona Macrae, "Tens of thousands of teenage girls believed to have fallen ill with debilitating illnesses after routine HPV cervical cancer jab," *Daily Mail*, June 1, 2015, http://www.dailymail.co.uk/health/article-3104629/Tens-thousands-teenage-girls-fall-ill-debilitating-illnesses-routine-HPV-cervical-cancer-jab.html#ixzz3cVNTcfQU.

313 David M. Reif et al., "Genetic Basis for Adverse Events Following Smallpox Vaccination," *Journal of Infectious Diseases* 198 (2008): 16–22, doi: 10.1086/588670.

314 See https://www.gdx.net/core/one-page-test-descriptions/TD_DetoxiGenomic_070313.pdf.

315 G.L. Arnold et al., "Plasma amino acids profiles in children with autism: Potential risk of nutritional deficiencies," *Journal of Autism and Developmental Disorders* 33 (2003): 449–454.

316 http://www.webmd.com/diabetes/alternative-medicine.

317 Koob, G. F. (1992) Drugs of abuse: anatomy, pharmacology and function of reward pathways.
 Trends in Pharmacological Sciences 13, 177–184.

318 Di Chiara, G. (1995) The role of dopamine in drug abuse viewed from the perspective of its role in motivation. Drug and Alcohol Dependence 38. 95-137.

319 White, F. J. (1996) Synaptic regulation of mesocorticolimbic dopamine neurons. Annual Review of Neuroscience 19, 405–436.

320 Kalivas, P. W. (1993) Neurotransmitter regulation of dopamine neurons in the ventral tegmental area.
 Brain Research Reviews 18, 75–113.
 White, F. J. (1996) Synaptic regulation of mesocorticolimbic dopamine neurons. Annual Review of Neuroscience 19, 405–436.

321 Kelley, A. E., Stinus, L. and Iversen, S. D. (1980) Interaction between $\delta$-ala2-met-enkephalin, A10 dopaminergic neurons and spontaneous behavior in the rat. Behavioral Brain Research1, 3–34.

322 Bozarth, M. A. and Wise, R. A. (1987) A psychomotor stimulant theory of addiction. Psychological Review 94, 469–492.

323 Mueller C.A., et al. (2015) High-dose baclofen for the treatment of alcohol dependence (BACLAD study): A randomized, placebo-controlled trial. European Neuropsychopharmacology
 25: 8, 1167-1177

324 Franklin, TR. Et al. (2010)_ The GABA B agonist baclofen reduces cigarette consumption in a preliminary double-blind placebo-controlled smoking reduction study. Drug Alcohol Depend. 2009 Jul 1; 103(1-2): 30–36.

325 Yanhua R., et al. (2009) J Neurosci. Cannabidiol, a nonpsychotropic component of cannabis, inhibits cue-induced heroin-seeking and normalizes discrete mesolimbic neuronal disturbances. 25:29(47), 14764-14769.

326 Michael Saulino, M., Jacobs, B.W. (2006) The pharmacological management of spasticity. J Neurosci Nurs. 38(6):456-459. Available at https://www.medscape.com/viewarticle/552267_3.

327 http://www.lifeextension.com/magazine/2008/5/D-Ribose-Energize-Your-Heart-Save-Your-Life/Page-01.

328 Aminocare Products L.P., aminocare.com.

329 K. M. Galalae, "The Subversion of Medicine and Public Health by International Security Prerogatives," *Epidemiology* (Sunnyvale) 5 (2015): 208. doi:10.4172/2161–1165.1000208.

330 N. Hovdenak and K. Haram, "Influence of mineral and vitamin supplements on pregnancy outcome," *European Journal of Obstetrics and Gynecology and Reproductive Biology* 164 (2012): 127–32, doi: 10.1016/j.ejogrb.2012.06.020.

331 X.M. Wang, H.Y. Wu, and X.J. Qiu, "Methylenetetrahydrofolate Reductase (*MTHFR*) Gene C677T Polymorphism and Risk of Preeclampsia: An Updated Meta-analysis Based on 51 Studies," *Archives of Medical Research* 44 (2013): 159–168, doi: 10.1016/j.arcmed.2013.01.011.

332 Ryan Grim, Matt Sledge, and Matt Ferner, "Key Figures In CIA-Crack Cocaine Scandal Begin To Come Forward," *Huffington Post*, October 10, 2014, http://www.huffingtonpost.com/2014/10/10/gary-webb-dark-alliance_n_5961748.html.

333 Jeanne Lenzer, "Majority of panelists on controversial new cholesterol guideline have current or recent ties to drug manufacturers," *BMJ* 347 (2013): f6989, doi: http://dx.doi.org/10.1136/bmj.f6989.

334 Milanda Rout, "Vioxx maker Merck and Co drew up doctor hit list," *Australian*, April 1, 2009, http://www.theaustralian.com.au/news/drug-company-drew-up-doctor-hit-list/story-e6frg6n6–1225693586492.

# Acknowledgments

The author would like to thank J. Mutter, Institute for Environmental Medicine and Hospital Epidemiology, University Hospital, Freiburg, Germany; Boyd Haley, Emeritus Professor of Chemistry at the University of Kentucky; and Lujene Clark of NoMercury for sharing their expertise.

I would also like to thank Skyhorse for printing a fairly heretical book written by someone who does not have a large media footprint and may never have one.

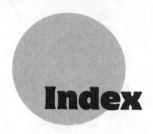

# Index

This is a truncated index as all drug names have been left out to conserve space. For example, I mention the drug Alinia thirty-eight times in the book, so perhaps this is a good place to point out I have no stock or other conflict of interest with the makers of Alinia. It is just a very beneficial drug.

5-HTP, 150
23&ME test, 145–146

**A**

A-10, 157–158
Acquired flaccid paralysis (AFP), 35–36, 46
Acrodynia, 112
Acute lymphocytic leukemia, 43
Adrenal fatigue, 162
Alcohol, 149
Alpha-ketoglutarate, 155
Alpha-lipoic acid (ALA), 154
Aluminum, 64–65, 92–93
Alzheimer's disease (AD), 8, 17, 29–30, 33, 35, 36, 59
Amalgam, 110–112, 161–163
American Academy of Pediatrics (AAP), 119–122
Amyloid plaques, 9, 60
Amyotrophic lateral sclerosis (ALS), 36–37, 58, 60
Animal Disease Center, 14–15
Antioxidants, 154
Arginine, 150
Arthritis, 61, 89–90
Astroturf organizations, 57
Attkisson, Sharyl, 57

Autism, 96–99, 100–101, 116–117, 118, 119–121, 128–130, 147
Autoimmunity, 115–116

**B**

Bacteria, beneficial, 154–155
Bantry Bay, 95–96
Bay Area, 10
Bees, 55, 62
Betaine hydrochloride, 154
Big Pharma, 174–177
Bill and Melinda Gates Foundation, 123
Biofilm, 19
Biomarkers, 24–25, 144, 147–148
Biosemiotics, 92–93
Bioweapons, 14–15
Bird flu, 133–134
Blood-brain barrier, 72–75
Blood supply, 12
Blood tests, 4–6
Blumenthal, Richard, 14
Boron, 151
*Borrelia burgdorferi*, 4
*Borrelia hermsii*, 4
Boxer, Barbara, 46–47
Brain injury, 76–85
Brazil, 51
Bronner, E. H., 73–74

Burgdorfer, Willy, 3–4
Butterfly, 64

**C**

C-8, 37
Calcium, 152
Cancer, cervical, 135–138
Caprylic acid, 66–67
Cardiovascular assessment, 147–148
Carnitine, 150
Carnosine, 150
Carson, Rachel, 43
CD 57, 24–25
CDC. *See* Centers for Disease Control
    and Prevention (CDC)
Centers for Disease Control and
    Prevention (CDC), 5, 10, 99–100
Cervical cancer, 135–138
Chan, Margaret, 139
Chelation, 161–162
Chemtrails, 65, 93–95
Chisso Corporation, 96
Chlorella, 155
Chromium, 152
Chronic fatigue syndrome, 61
Chronic traumatic encephalopathy (CTE),
    76–85
CIA, 93–94
Cigarettes, 137
Clotting genomics, 146
Cockburn, Alexander, 107–108
Coconut oil, 66–67
Coenzyme Q10, 154
Colony collapse disorder (CCD), 55, 62–63
Conflicts of interest, 13
Consensus, 55
Contraceptive vaccines, 106–109
Controversy, 3–4, 10
Cook, Ken, 38
Copper, 42, 60, 152
Cowden Protocol, 18
Creutzfeldt-Jakob disease (CJD), 42
Crichton, Michael, 55
Crohn's disease (CD), 68–72
Cruciferous vegetables, 136–137

Curcumin, 60
Cysteine, 114
Cytochrome P450 2D6, 59
Cytokine storm, 20–23

**D**

Danish population studies, 101–102,
    116–117
DDE (dichlorodiphenyldichloroethylene),
    30–33
DDT, 33–37, 49–50
Dearborn criteria, 4–6
Dementia, 29–54
Dental amalgam, 110–112, 161–162
Detoxification, 52–54, 155–156, 158–160
Detoxification genomics, 146
Diagnosis, of Lyme, 4–6, 11–12, 15–16
Diagnostics, 145–147
Dicofol, 33, 51
Diet, 19, 22, 45–60, 53, 136–137, 148–149
Digestive enzymes, 154
Diphtheria, 126
Drinking water, 44, 73–75
Drug reps, 176–177

**E**

Ebola, 142
Ebsen, Buddy, 92–93
Endocrine-disrupting chemicals, 40
Endogenous/exogenous retrovirus (ERV),
    87–88
Environmental law, 59–60
Environmental Protection Agency (EPA),
    63–64
Epidemiological studies, 116–117
Epigallocatechin gallate (ECCG), 133–134
Epsom salt, 155
Epstein-Barr virus (EBV), 16, 17, 23, 37, 86
Essential fatty acids (EFAs), 157
Ethylmercury, 113–115
Evidence-based medicine, 8–9

**F**

Fetal alcohol syndrome, 76–85
Fillings, dental, 110–112, 161–162

Fleming, Alexander, 91
Fluoride, 72–75
Flu vaccine, 132–133
Folinic acid, 155
Food, 19, 45–60, 136–137, 148–149
Food allergies, 73
Football, 80–83
Fruit, 148

**G**

Gamma-aminobenzoic acid (GABA), 150
Garlic, 25
Gastritis, 55–56
Genetically modified organisms (GMOs), 38
Genetic testing, 145–147
Georgia Guidestones, 94, 95
Gerberding, Julie, 97
Glutathione (GSH), 53, 114, 150–151
Glutathione S-transferases (GSTs), 52–53
Gluten, 22, 149
Glyphosate, 38–42, 45, 72–73
Graham, David J., 123
Grains, 149
Great Plains Diagnostics, 147
Green tea, 54, 133–134
Gulf War, 58, 61
Gut dysbiosis, 72–75

**H**

H1NI virus, 131–132, 133–134
H5N1 virus, 133–134
*Haemophilus influenzae,* 127
Harch, Paul, 80–81
Heavy metals, 159
*Heliobacter pylori,* 55–56
Hensley, Charles, 134
Hepatitis B, 127–128
Herbs, 25–26, 148
Herx reaction, 20–23
Hib vaccine, 127
Hideyo, Noguchi, 9
HIV, 86–87
Homeless population, 27
HPV vaccine, 135–139, 140
HTLV, 58

Human chorionic gonadotropin (hCG), 108
Human endogenous retrovirus-K, 58–59
Human gamma retrovirus (HGRV), 87
Hyperbaric oxygen treatment, 3, 76–85, 88, 89–90
Hypericum, 53

**I**

IGeneX, 15–16
IgG, 16–17
IgM, 16–17
Immune genomics, 146–147
Immune support, 155
Indole-3-carbinol (I3C), 136–137, 155
Infant mortality, 123–124
Infectious Disease Society of America (IDSA), 12–14
Infectious disease testing, 148
Inflammatory bowel disease (IBD), 68–75
Inflammatory reaction, 20–23
Influenza vaccine, 132–133
Inositol hexaphosphate (IP6), 157
Institute of Medicine (IOM), 103–104
Intelligence, 92
Iron, 153

**J**

Jarisch-Herxheimer reaction, 20–23
Johnston, Dick, 119

**K**

Katz, Emily, 46–47
Keratin, 27–28
Klinghardt Protocol, 18

**L**

Law, environmental, 59–60
Lawrence, D. H., 75
Lee, Sin Hang, 139
Leukemia, 43
Lewy bodies, 59
Licorice, 156
Lincoln, Abraham, 177
Lipid genomics, 146
Lithium, 153

Lou Gehrig's disease, 36–37, 58
Lyme disease
    experience with, 2
    prevalence of, 10
    treatment of, 17–20, 88–89
Lymphoma, 37, 41–42

**M**
MacDonald, Alan B., 9
Mad cow disease, 42–45
Magnesium, 153
Malaria, 173
Maney, Patt, 84
Manganese, 24, 42, 153
Marshall, Barry J., 55–56
Mastic gum, 56
Measles, 70. *See also* MMR vaccine
Meats, 149
Melatonin, 157
Meningitis, 127, 140–141
Mercury, 91–122, 160–164
Metals, heavy, 160
Methylcobalamine, 156
Methylmercury, 113–114
Methylsulfonylmethane (MSM), 151
Microcephaly, 51–52
Micronutrients, 53
Minamata Convention on Mercury, 111
Minamata disease, 95–96
MMR vaccine, 88, 100, 123, 128–131
Mojab, Ryan, 128
Molybdenum, 153
Monarch butterfly, 64
Monolaurin, 154
Morgellons disease, 27–28
Morrison, David, 108
Multiple sclerosis (MS), 79–80, 85–88, 88–89
Mumps. *See* MMR vaccine
*Mycobacterium avium paratuberculosis* (MAP), 69
Mycoplasma, 61
Mycoplasma multiplex PCR detection, 148

**N**
N-acetyl cysteine (NAC), 152
National Football League (NFL), 80–83
Ndumbe, Peter, 107
Neonicotinoids, 63
Neurodegenerative disease, 58
Neurodevelopmental disorders, 43
Newby, Kris, 14
9/11 attacks, 57
Non-Hodgkin's lymphoma (NHL), 37, 41–42
Nutrition, 19, 45–60, 53, 136–137, 148–149
Nutritional biomarkers, 147–148
Nuts, 149

**O**
Omega 3s, 88
Oregano, 25
Orwell, George, 29
Oxytocin, 157

**P**
Parkinson's disease (PD), 59–60
Peptic ulcer disease, 55–56
Perfluorooctanoic, 37
Pertussis, 126–127
Pharmaceutical companies, 9–10, 55–56, 61, 174–177
Phenyl butyrate, 157–158
Philippines, 108
Pink disease, 112
Pirkle, Jim, 91–92
Plato, 171
Plum Island, 14–15
Poling, Hannah, 96–99
Poliomyelitis, 47–48, 125–126
Polychlorinated biphenyl (PCB), 37
Polymerase chain reaction (PCR), 15
Population control, 105, 106, 130
Powassan virus, 26
Preeclampsia (PEE), 173–174
Prions, 42–45, 60
Probiotics, 153–154

Profits, 9–10
Proteolytic enzymes, 21
Protocols, 18–19
Pyridoxal-5-phosphate, 156

**R**
Rappoport, John, 130
Ravenholt, Reimart, 108
Regulation, 44
Reporting, 12–13
Resveratrol, 154–155
Rheumatoid arthritis (RA), 61, 89–90
Ribose, 157
Rocky Mountain Spotted Fever, 22
Roman Empire, 172
Ross & Brooke Successful Treatment
    Recipe, 18
Roundup, 39, 45
Rubella. *See* MMR vaccine
Russell, Bertrand, 99

**S**
S-adenosylmethionine (SAM-e), 53–54,
    152
Salt & Vitamin C Protocol, 18
San Francisco Bay Area, 10
Schizophrenia, 31, 33
Selenium, 152
Semmelweiss, Ignaz, 160
September 11 attacks, 57
Serratiopeptidase, 21
*Silent Spring* (Carson), 43
Sloppy-stool syndrome, 21
Smoking, 137
Spices, 149
Spirochaetaceae, 5
Starfield, Barbara, 68
Steere, Allen, 6
Steinberg, Darrell, 47
Stock, Alfred, 110
Stratospheric Aerosol Geoengineering, 65
Stratospheric aerosol injection (SAI),
    93–95
Streptococcal antibody panel, 148
Substance abuse, 176

Sugar, 19, 149
Supplements, 53, 150–158
Swine flu, 131–132, 133–134
Syphilis, 9, 11

**T**
Tacaribe virus, 26
Taurine, 151
TDP-43, 59
Tea
    black, 134–135
    green, 54, 133–134
    white sage, 21–22
Teflon, 37
TENDR, 43–44
Tetanus, 108, 126
Theaflavin, 134–135
Thimerosal, 97–98, 101, 104–105,
    112–113, 114–115, 116–117, 119–122
Thompson, William, 100–101, 130
Thorsen, Poul, 101–102, 103
Tick population, 26
Ticks, 2, 6–8
Tics, 101
Tolstoy, Leo, 1
Traumatic brain injury, 76–85
Treatment, of Lyme disease, 17–20
Trench fever, 27
*Treponema pallidum*, 9
Tropical spastic paraparesis (TSP), 58
Tuberculosis, 11

**U**
Ulcerative colitis, 68–69

**V**
Vaccines, 70, 96–109. *See also* Autism;
    Thimerosal
    diphtheria, 126
    endogenous/exogenous viruses in, 87–88
    flu, 132–133
    hepatitis B, 127–128
    Hib, 127
    HPV, 135–139, 140
    infant mortality and, 123–124

for Lyme, 6–8
meningitis, 140–141
MMR, 88, 100, 123, 128–131
pertussis, 126–127
polio, 125–126
tetanus, 126
Vaccine safety data, 103–109
Vanadium, 153
Vismara, Louis, 47–49
Vitamin A, 53, 156–157
Vitamin C, 157
Vitamin D, 134, 137, 156
Vitamin E, 157
Vitamin K, 157
Vitamins, 156–157

**W**
Water, 44, 73–75
Weil, Bill, 113

Western blot, 4–6, 15
White sage tea, 21–22
*Wizard of Oz* (film), 93
Wolf-Dieter Storl Protocol, 18

**X**
X-linked severe combined
    immunodeficiency (X-SCID), 87

**Y**
Yeast, 23–24
Yenshu, Emmanuel, 107

**Z**
Zika virus, 50–52, 141–142
Zinc, 153